Praise for Essence of

"As one of our preeminent tarot scholars and teachers, Mary K. Greer has done it again. In *Essence of Tarot*, Greer unearths new levels of detail and outlines accessible ways to connect with your tarot deck. Whether you are brand new in developing your tarot practice or decades in, you'll find that Greer effortlessly engages with her audience and reminds us all of the magic within that tarot can help unlock. I consider Mary K. Greer to be my tarot fairy godmother, and I'm delighted for her to become yours."

—Rachel True, author of *True Heart Intuitive Tarot*

"Mary K. Greer is to tarot what BTS is to K-Pop. Her name has become synonymous with tarot and with good reason. For several decades, she has established herself as both a leading authority and a pioneer, transforming the way many approach tarot today. In *Essence of Tarot*, Greer once again proves why she remains one of the most respected voices in the field. Drawing from her deep tarot knowledge, she skillfully integrates essential oils and ritual practices, bringing a fresh and innovative method to spiritual work. Greer offers practical and accessible advice for amplifying tarot readings through the use of scent and ritual. Whether you're just beginning with tarot or have been practicing for years, this book serves as an essential guide for those wanting to strengthen their bond with the cards, guided by one of tarot's most trusted and knowledgeable experts."

—Mat Auryn, author of *The Psychic Art of Tarot*,
Psychic Witch, and *Mastering Magick*

"There are some books that hold a special place on my bookshelf. Many of these have been out of print for some time, which makes them irreplaceable. *Essence of Tarot* (previously *The Essence of Magic: Tarot, Ritual and Aromatherapy*) by Mary K. Greer is one such book. Thankfully, it's back in print! With illustrated charts and detailed information, this beloved book masterfully blends the worlds of tarot, aromatherapy, and ritual magic. Whether you're a seasoned practitioner or a curious beginner, Greer's insights into the use of essential oils for divination, meditation, and spiritual practices will deepen your craft. Her expert knowledge on the alchemical properties of herbs and oils, alongside practical tarot interpretations, make this an indispensable guide for anyone seeking to enrich their magickal journey. A must-have for your metaphysical library! While I'll never part with my original copy, I'm delighted to make space for this new edition."

—Theresa Reed, author of *The Cards You're Dealt:*
How to Deal When Life Gets Real (A Tarot Guidebook)

"Pamela Colman Smith, the visionary artist behind the Waite-Smith deck, possessed the gift of synesthesia, transforming sound into vivid, mystical imagery. In *Essence of Tarot*, a landmark work, now at last republished, Mary K. Greer transcends yet another sensory frontier, inviting us into the world of sacred fragrance—where the scent of oils unveils secret correspondences and deepens the mysteries embedded within the tarot. This extraordinary book offers a transformative approach to engaging with the cards, nose first. One that will resonate profoundly with many, reaffirming tarot as a magical and deeply sensual art form. Greer's unparalleled legacy continues to illuminate our path, inspiring a reimagining of tarot as a multisensory tool."

—Laetitia Barbier, author of *Tarot and Divination Cards:*
A Visual Archive

"To me, Mary K. Greer is the undisputed Queen of Tarot; much of what I learned for my own practice came from her books. So you can imagine my excitement when she combined tarot with two of my other favorites—rituals and essential oils. This book takes the tarot to the next level, and I for one can't wait to try out many of the treasures that lie inside."

—Deborah Blake, author of *Everyday Witch Tarot*
and *Everyday Witchcraft*

"Brimming with magic, *Essence of Tarot* teaches the reader to harness the supernatural power of their olfactory senses by combining plant energies with tarot archetypes. This process results in a deeply intuitive system of manifestation and psychic pathworking. Mary K. Greer's masterful work belongs on every tarotist's bookshelf!"

—Sasha Graham, author of *365 Tarot Spreads* and *Dark Wood Tarot*

"When I first began making zodiacal perfumes several years ago, I was able to briefly borrow a library copy of this book (then titled *The Essence of Magic*), and was dismayed to learn I could not find one to purchase! So as a tarot reader, maker of correspondence-based scents, and longtime admirer of Mary Greer and all her works, I feel a great injustice has been remedied in the republication of *Essence of Tarot*. Mary's scent-note correspondences for the major and minor arcanas are thoughtful and research-based, yet also imaginative—an indispensable resource for any practitioner who lives by the creed 'As above, so below.'"

—T. Susan Chang, author of *The Living Tarot*
and creator of the Tarotista perfume line on Etsy

"This stunning tarot herbal book magically connects tarot and essential oils, guiding us to connect with the elemental forces within each card. Pure enchantment."

—Liz Dean, author of *The Ultimate Guide to Tarot*

"*Essence of Tarot* is a true treasure for any reader looking to deepen their experience with the tarot. It masterfully combines the sacred art of essential oils, magic, and rituals with the world of tarot. It allows you to extend your knowledge and understanding of the cards in a way that truly engages the senses. Mary masterfully guides you through the pages of this book, brings her legendary tarot experience and weaves it together with the world of practical enchantment. Whether you're a seasoned tarot reader or just beginning your journey, this book will open new doors of insight, clarity, and empowerment in your readings. A must-have for anyone who seeks to bring more intention and magic into their practice."

—Ethony Dawn, author of *Tarot Grimoire*

"Unlike our visual and auditory senses, which we perceive after lots of processing between the sense organs and the brain, the sense of smell is far more immediate—almost like a direct hit of sensation that triggers emotions, memories, and meanings. Mary K. Greer weaves together this powerful agent of smell with the metaphors and symbolism of the tarot to deliver a heady concoction. Contextualizing the work with science, sociopolitics, and the history of olfaction along with tarot and astrological correspondences and symbolism, *Essence of Tarot* is alchemy at its best with new insights blooming with every card and herb. As a neuroscientist, I use the scientific method a lot to approach the world—but also recognize there is wealth of cultural and historical knowledge on the power of herbs and essential oils that has been passed down through lore, practical medicine, and wisdom of elders. Mary has carefully curated this wealth of herbal wisdom and layered it with the depth of meaning from the tarot. While humans are primarily visual, a lot of our intuitive processing relies on unconscious inputs from other senses. *Essence of Tarot* is a sensual pleasure of a book and will truly open up your practice by moving from beyond just the visual realm, creating a more holistic, insightful experience."

—Siddharth Ramakrishnan, PhD, neuroscientist
and author of *The Neuroscience of Tarot*

"What happens when the world's preeminent tarot scholar performs literary alchemy and creates a book that adeptly blends ritual, tarot, and the magic of essential oils? You get Mary K. Greer's *Essence of Tarot*. For those of us who have longed for a copy of this out-of-print book, this freshly updated and retitled edition is pure inspiration. *Essence of Tarot* covers the foundations of magical aromatherapy and tarot for those who need a refresher as well as giving correspondences and deep magical plant lore that opens up dozens of creative possibilities for spellcasters of any experience level. I am sure that, like me, you will refer to this book again and again for new, inventive ways to make even more magic with your tarot deck."

—Madame Pamita, author of *Magical Tarot*

"Mary K. Greer is a leader and one of our greatest teachers in the tarot community. Her knowledge and expertise are invaluable. In *Essence of Tarot*, Mary clearly defines and lays out the power of scent. We learn how scent in combination with the energies of the tarot can create and call in support for internal transformation for movement forward. One of the greatest lessons learned is how scent combined with imagination and ritual creates action, which in turn creates magic. Mary shares tarot oils, rituals, affirmations, and tarot spreads to guide us forward. *Essence of Tarot* opens up new ways and options for the tarot world to explore. A must-read for all tarot enthusiasts."

—Ailynn Halvorson, author of *The Tarot Apothecary*

"One of the most important of Mary K. Greer's books has returned after being unavailable for far too long. A superbly useful, delightfully readable, and skillful melding of use of scent applied to the practice of tarot, *Essence of Tarot* offers a treasure trove of practical information that many practitioners will soon consider a warm and helpful addition to their toolbox. When this book initially came out, it broke new ground in what could be done with both aromatherapy and divination, and with her knack for meticulous research, fearless exploration, and warmly accessible prose, Mary opened new doors of possibilities. In the years since the book was first published, aromatherapy has become almost ubiquitous, but this book remains unique and beneficial. A must-have for every diviner's shelf!"

—Thalassa, creatrix of the San Francisco Bay Area
Tarot Symposium (SF BATS)

"Mary Greer has a true gift that shines through all her writing. It's her ability to understand the power of tarot that guides us on our physical and spiritual paths and eases us through emotional situations. In *Essence of Tarot*, she also taps into the healing aspects of aromatherapy and its use of aromatic plants and essential oils. Her intuitive sense of using both tarot and aromatherapy for personal transformation creates the perfect marriage. Greer artfully blends these two healing arts together as she guides the reader into fascinating new dimensions of tarot that you will want to add to your skillset. I especially love the clear writing style and attention to detail to the history, symbolism, and creative uses of tarot and aromas. The result is a very unique book that will open new doors into your appreciation of tarot."

—Kathi Keville, director of American Herb Association and
author of *Aromatherapy: A Complete Guide to the Healing Art*,
and *Essential Oils and Aromatherapy for Dummies*

Essence of Tarot

Using Essential Oils, Magic & Rituals to Empower Your Readings

Mary K. Greer

FOREWORD BY
JUDIKA ILLES

WEISER BOOKS

*This book is dedicated to my Kneebone family:
Casi, Dave, Eli and Clara.
May the essence of magic always be yours.*

This edition first published in 2025 by Weiser Books, an imprint of Red Wheel/Weiser, LLC
With offices at:
65 Parker Street, Suite 7
Newburyport, MA 01950
www.redwheelweiser.com

Copyright © 2025 by Mary K. Greer
Foreword by Judika Illes © 2025 by Red Wheel/Weiser, LLC

All rights reserved. No part of this publication may be reproduced or transmitted in any form or by any means, electronic or mechanical, including photocopying, recording, or by any information storage and retrieval system, without permission in writing from Red Wheel/Weiser, LLC. Reviewers may quote brief passages. Previously published in 1993 as *The Essence of Magic* by Newcastle Publishing Company, Inc., ISBN 0-87877-180-8.

ISBN: 978-1-57863-852-9

Library of Congress Cataloging-in-Publication Data

Names: Greer, Mary K. (Mary Katherine) author. | Illes, Judika, writer of
foreword.
Title: The essence of tarot : using essential oils, magic, and rituals to empower your readings /
Mary K. Greer ; foreword by Judika Illes.
Description: Newburyport, MA : Weiser Books, 2025. | Includes bibliographical references. |
Summary: "The ancient art of perfumery and fragrance have long been a component of magical
and spiritual rituals. This book demonstrates how this primordial art can be used to enhance
modern tarot practices, whether for divination, meditation, or affirmations. Learn how to create
a more magical life through the union of tarot and aromatherapy"-- Provided by publisher.
Identifiers: LCCN 2024042276 | ISBN 9781578638529 (trade paperback) | ISBN 9781633413504
(ebook)
Subjects: LCSH: Tarot. | Essences and essential oils. | Magic. | Ritual. | BISAC: BODY, MIND &
SPIRIT / Divination / Tarot | BODY, MIND & SPIRIT /Occultism
Classification: LCC BF1879.T2 G7193 2025 | DDC
133.3/2424--dc23/eng/20241017
LC record available at https://lccn.loc.gov/2024042276

Cover and interior design by Brittany Craig
Typeset in Cormorant Garamond

Printed in the United States of America
IBI
10 9 8 7 6 5 4 3 2 1

This book contains advice and information relating to herbs and essential oils and is not meant to diagnose, treat, or prescribe. It should be used to supplement, not replace, the advice of your physician or other trained healthcare practitioner. If you know or suspect you have a medical condition, are experiencing physical symptoms, or if you feel unwell, seek your physician's advice before embarking on any medical program or treatment. Readers using the information in this book do so entirely at their own risk, and the author and publisher accept no liability if adverse effects are caused.

Contents

List of Charts and Tables . . . . *x*

Foreword, by Judika Illes . . . . *xi*

Acknowledgments . . . . *xv*

Introduction *1*

1. Essential Oils 3

   Introduction *3*

   What Are Essential Oils? *4*

   Extraction Techniques *6*

   The Sense of Smell *7*

   The Sociopolitics of Essence *11*

2. A Magical History of Oils 15

   Earliest Uses *15*

   Alchemy *33*

3. About the Tarot 37

   Basic Information *37*

   History *38*

   The Law of Correspondence *40*

   Oils and Scents as Symbols *41*

4. Imagination and Aroma Imaging 51

   The Nature of Olfaction *51*

   Aroma and Imagination *54*

   Aroma Imaging with Tarot Oils *54*

   The Tarot Oils *57*

5.	The Tarot Oils	59
	Astrological Correspondences	59
	Choosing the Oils to Work With	62
	The Major Arcana Tarot Oils	63
	The Minor Arcana Essence Oils	111
6.	Magic and Ritual	115
	Making Magic	115
	About Rituals	117
	Outline for Ritual	120
	The Magical Forms of Essential Oils	125
7.	Tarot Oil Techniques	131
	Grounding and Centering Process	132
	Communicating with a Plant	133
	Communicating with an Essential Oil	134
	Making and Using Tarot Oils	135
	Steps for Charging and Making Tarot Oils	140
	Consecrating Your Tarot Oils	142
	Anointing Yourself with Oil	144
	Uses for the Tarot Oils	146
	Using Affirmations with Tarot Oils	152
	Ritual Uses for Tarot Cards and Oils	153
8.	Tarot Spreads	159
	The Quintessence Spread	159
	The Creative Work-Cycle Spread	162
	The Magic Spread	163

Appendixes

A. The Lifetime and Year Cards.......................... 166

  The Personality and Soul Cards................................ 166

  Determining Your Personality and Soul Cards 168

  The Hidden Factor Card...................................... 169

  Determining Your Hidden Factor Card............................173

  The Year Card(s)..173

  Determining Your Year Card(s) 174

B. Master Chart of the Essential Oils..................... 175

  Notes.. 181

  Bibliography.. 187

List of Charts and Tables

Minor Arcana Suits Chart 38

Table of Tarot Correspondences. 42

Astrological Correspondences: Elements, Planets,
and Signs 60

Astrological Rulerships and Oppositions 62

The 22 Major Arcana Tarot Oils. 64

Important Warnings 65

Major Arcana Substitutions for Minor Arcana
Cards 112

The 56 Minor Arcana Essence Oils 113

Table of Planetary "Hours" 139

Patterns of Personal Destiny 170

Master Chart of the Essential Oils 175

Foreword

It was 1966. I was six years old, and my sister was a freshman at Cooper Union, a college located in New York City's East Village. She was gone all day, and I genuinely just missed her, but, in addition, I eagerly awaited her nightly return for other, ulterior reasons. She frequently came home bearing treasure.

Sometimes it was music in the form of record albums, but often it was books and usually those books were metaphysical ones. At that time, the Samuel Weiser bookshop, among the finest purveyors of esoterica in the world, was situated near Cooper Union, and my sister would often shop there. One evening, she arrived home with tarot cards. As the old saying goes, "just one look is all it took." I was struck by the lightning bolt of love. To this day, that love has never wavered. My love for tarot remains true.

Similarly, I recall when and where I first encountered essential oils: 1988, Hoboken, New Jersey, where I was then living. I read a small magazine advertisement that suggested that these oils might be helpful for a minor physical concern I had. In response, I purchased a small bottle of essential oil of frankincense. I was not expecting magic, but once again, it was love at first sight—or in this case, at first smell. When I opened that bottle, it was as if a benevolent genie had emerged to enrich my life. As I experienced what frankincense could do—magically, spiritually, therapeutically—I was totally and permanently smitten.

My first encounter with Mary K. Greer's glorious book, then titled *The Essence of Magic*, would occur ten years later and on the other side of the continent. It was 1998, and I now lived in Los Angeles. At that time, I was studying essential oils earnestly, while simultaneously working as a professional tarot reader. I was also pursuing research that would eventually find its way into my book, *Encyclopedia of 5,000 Spells*, although it was then only for my own use and personal pleasure.

I read everything I could find about essential oils, which could be frustrating as, at that time and with very few exceptions—such as Scott Cunningham's pioneering *Magical Aromatherapy*—most books focused exclusively on their therapeutic use. And then I found *The Essence of Magic*. Once again, that lightning bolt struck. I felt as if, with its blend of tarot, essential oils, and ritual, the author might have written the book especially for me. I suspect many others will feel the same. I fell in love with it upon first reading, and I may love it even more today.

Readers, treasure your books. If you see something that you want to read, please do it when the opportunity presents itself. It is a sad truth that so many wonderful books are put out of print for a vast variety of reasons, having nothing to do with the quality of the books themselves. Such was the fate of Mary's book on fragrance, tarot, and ritual, which languished out of print for years, the few remaining copies commanding exorbitant prices that made it prohibitively expensive to acquire. The publication of this new, retitled edition thus fills me with joy.

Essence of Tarot is a revolutionary book. Countless books are devoted to essential oils and countless more devoted to tarot, but *Essence of Tarot's* merger of the two is unique. Essential oils are *synergistic*, meaning that their combined effect is greater than the sum of their individual parts. In other words, essential oil of lavender has profound effects, as does essential oil of rosemary. But when blended, their combined impact (whether therapeutic or magical) is exponentially greater.

Essence of Tarot is synergistic, too. Tarot cards are powerful, as are essential oils. As Greer demonstrates in this book, when blended into a united practice, their effects provide us with exponentially more power. As she writes in this book, "Using both aroma and tarot together magically, as we shall see, gives us an incredibly powerful tool for personal growth, self-understanding, and for aligning ourselves with elemental forces that manifest in both the physical and metaphysical planes."

The ritual use of fragrance ranks among the oldest sacred and magical arts. Although tarot is comparatively modern, the art of divination itself is ancient. Both—sacred fragrance rituals and divination—are our common human heritage, belonging to us all.

I came to this book already familiar with tarot and essential oils, but that's not necessary. *Essence of Tarot* introduces essential oils to tarotists and tarot to aromatherapists. The author first discusses essential oils and how they are used. After taking us on a whirlwind tour of diverse historical traditions of sacred fragrance rituals, Greer provides an introduction to tarot in chapter 3. *Essence of Tarot* contains many beautiful rituals and recipes, as well as clear instructions for constructing rituals and creating tarot-themed oil blends.

Mary K. Greer is among the world's foremost authorities on tarot. Her mastery of essential oils and the magical art of fragrance may be less well known but probably not for long, as it radiates throughout the pages of *Essence of Tarot*. That said, for those new to essential oils and wishing to be prepared, let me give you a quick 101 recap:

Despite their name, essential oils are not true oils like olive oil or safflower oil. Essential oils are *not* oily; most are liquid and typically described as *watery*, although a few, such as vetiver, are more viscous. Essential oils are profound, powerful, *fragrant* plant extracts. Volatile liquids (meaning that they evaporate quickly), essential oils are extracted from aromatic plants by various methods. Their use dates back thousands of years: as a component of ancient Egypt's mummification process, for example. Modern aromatherapy, born in France in the mid-20th century, is the manipulation of essential oils for therapeutic, cosmetic, and ritual use, as well as for perfumery. This is its true, technical, and accurate definition, even though the word "aromatherapy" is frequently erroneously used to sell things like air fresheners.

Essential oils are highly concentrated. When it comes to their use, typically less is more. As actual plant extracts, they potentially exert a profound physical impact upon bodies. Essential oils should never be taken internally

Foreword

except under expert supervision. (French physicians, for example, prescribe and supervise their therapeutic use.) Nor should most essential oils be applied undiluted to the skin. Caution is advised if you are pregnant, trying to conceive, breast feeding, or are subject to various medical conditions. Certain essential oils are contraindicated for those with seizure disorders, for instance.

Their impact is also profoundly *metaphysical*. Essential oils have been described as the lifeblood of a plant, containing the plant's life essence. As this book demonstrates, they serve as a gateway to accessing the essence of divination systems, such as tarot; but also, most especially, they are a key to unlocking your own personal and unique magical powers, to discovering your own precious essence, empowering you, and furthering your own personal practices, whatever they might be.

Part of the revolutionary nature of *Essence of Tarot* is that by creating this synergy of tarot and essential oils, Mary offers us the possibility of extending this capacity for synergy even further. Essential oils are already a significant component of spell work. Perhaps you have a passion for runes, astrology, or numerology. Envision how the incorporation of essential oils can enhance these systems. The sky is the limit.

Reading *Essence of Tarot* is like entering a beautiful hothouse filled with exquisite flowers, divine aromas, and potent magical tools. As I write, it is now over twenty-five years since I first read the book. Since then, I have been privileged to meet and converse with Mary K. Greer, who is as brilliant and kind as *Essence of Tarot* suggests. Readers, savor these pages.

May they lead you to wonderful, safe, and happy destinations.

—Judika Illes, author of *Pure Magic,*
Encyclopedia of 5,000 Spells and other books
August 15, 2024, the Festival of Torches

Acknowledgments

I wish to thank Red Wheel/Weiser and especially Judika Illes for her assistance and support in getting this book updated and back in print. I also want to acknowledge the inspiration I received from aromatherapists Kathi Keville and Victoria Edwards and from the years I attended and taught at the Women's Herbal Gatherings in Oregon and Northern California.

Introduction

Are you already familiar with tarot? Or were you drawn here by an interest in the sensory aspects of ritual and magic? Perhaps it was the therapeutic qualities of essential oils? What you'll discover is these three complement each other through a shared emphasis on symbolism, intention, and the active pursuit of self-knowledge.

The tarot deck serves as a powerful tool for divination, self-reflection, and guidance, offering a visual and symbolic language through which you can access hidden truths, gain insights, and explore possibilities. Its most important purpose is to help you meet whatever comes in the best possible way. Aromatherapy is the practice of using essential oils and aromatic plant extracts to promote physical, emotional, and spiritual well-being. Combining these with magical rituals creates a multidimensional sensory experience that deepens a connection to the cards, the elemental spirits, and the energies you seek to invoke. By harnessing the power of intention, symbolism, and energy, you can amplify your desire and focus, imbuing the divinatory process with a sense of reverence, soul purpose, and potency. Engaging the senses stimulates the imagination and deepens a connection to supernatural realms. Tarot provides a map, marked by symbols, to show the way; while ritual is symbolism in action.

Integrating the visual symbolism of tarot cards, the soul force of essential oils, and the directed focus of magical rituals, you can create a transformative and immersive experience for spiritual exploration and personal growth.

We'll begin our journey by becoming familiar with some of the spiritual, magical, and healing practices associated with the plants and essential oils that have been used in traditional cultures for millennia.

CHAPTER 1

Essential Oils

*"Who that has reason, and his smell,
Would not among roses and jasmine dwell,
Rather than all his spirits choke
With exhalations of dirt and smoke?"*
—Abraham Cowley, 17th-century poet

Introduction

Fragrance has been associated with mystery, magic, and sorcery for as long as we know—from the earliest orally transmitted myths up to the most recent book on essential oils or perfumes, which inevitably finds the author waxing poetically about the "bewitching" qualities of scent. Edwin Morris, in *Fragrance: The Story of Perfume from Cleopatra to Chanel*, tells us how he became interested in the subject: "The wizardry of the sense of olfaction proved so intriguing . . . The more I studied the historical records, the more I saw that in all major civilizations fragrance was a cultural need associated with magic, pleasure and even healing and therapy."[1]

Part of the mystery comes from the fact that we perceive the presence of essential oils but cannot see them. Scent works invisibly. Apothecaries of old called essential oils "spirits," not only because they were nonmaterial like heavenly spirits but also because they had mysterious effects on people. And yet, essence (which comes from the Latin *esse*, "to be, to exist") refers to what is actual or real, reflecting the truth that mystery is at the heart of reality. The word oil itself is from Latin *olere*, "to emit a smell" (from the Greek root for olive). Thus, essential oils literally mean something like "fragrant spiritual substances." Essential oils are called volatile, from the Latin *volare* (meaning "to fly" or "wings"), because they soar and are so fleeting. The Germans call them *ätherische Öl*, "ethereal oil"—for ethereal means "of the celestial spheres; heavenly, unearthly; spiritual."

As Diane Ackerman points out in *A Natural History of the Senses*, even though we smell with every breath, it is a mute sense, for we have no vocabulary to describe how something smells to someone who hasn't smelled it. "Smells are often right on the tip of our tongues—but no closer," she says, "and it gives them a kind of magical distance, a mystery, a power without a name, a sacredness."[2] Fragrance is not entirely a physical substance. One can scent a large room for ten years with a tiny piece of musk and yet there will be no loss in its weight.

On the other hand, the germ-killing power of several essential oils is outstanding; thyme being twelve times more powerful than carbolic acid. Clove is nine times stronger, while even cinnamon and rose are seven times stronger, and rosemary and lavender follow closely. Cinnamon essential oil kills the typhoid bacillus in about twelve minutes, while clove and geranium take only a little longer. Hippocrates is said to have freed Athens from the plague by using fumigations of aromatic plants. And perfumers generally throughout Europe have remained immune to infectious bacterial diseases.

Essential oils are powerful yet ethereal, perceptible yet nonmaterial. They are fleeting, yet they linger.

What Are Essential Oils?

Essential oils are the concentrated essences of plants and flowers—their soul stuff. They directly affect your vital force and are therefore very powerful. A small amount—often only one drop—goes a long way and operates quickly.

These are not inert, dead substances. Through photosynthesis, plants take the energy of sunlight and of the cosmos itself, the energy of the earth, and the exhaled life force of humans and animals and transform them into various new forms. But this vital energy is concentrated and efficiently stored in essential oils, which is why they have been called "liquid light." Because they work simultaneously on the body, mind, and spirit, all three of these effects must be taken into account when using an essential oil.

It was through alchemy, the medieval art and science of spiritual transformation, that the secret of extracting scents in concentrated form—from flowers, herbs, spices, and trees (using their blossoms, leaves, barks, roots, woods, resins, fruits, and seeds)—was found. According to anthroposophist Franz Hartmann, it is the molecules of essential oil that contain the most profound healing properties: "The medical virtues of plants are in the ethereal particles, which act upon the life-ethers with which they are in affinity, and so set up vibrations in certain corresponding nerve-currents and organs in the human and animal body. . . . [When] diluted or 'etherealized' the action is then not merely physical or mechanical, but is metaphysical, because it involves the active life principle and Consciousness."[3] Plant oils, being fatty, are also storehouses of warmth provided by nature and possess a natural biological affinity to the metabolic processes of human beings.

Essential oils can now be readily purchased in most health-food stores or via mail order. They are usually designated as "pure, natural" versus "fragrance oils" that contain synthetics. Because essential oils are produced in a variety of ways and "grades," and because the plants and flowers grow in different countries all over the world, their prices vary greatly: true rose oil may cost fifty to one hundred times as much as orange or tangerine oil. Prices also vary from year to year, depending on the natural and political climate of the regions in which they are grown and produced.

There is a big difference between "true, natural" essential oils and those fragrances that contain synthetics. Don't be fooled. Most jasmine oils sold in stores for under ten dollars contain little or no true jasmine essential oil. A

Essential Oils

quarter-million hand-picked blossoms—which take an experienced picker about twenty days to gather—yield one ounce of jasmine oil. Synthetics may be okay for everyday wear, but for magical and healing purposes they do not have the vital life force required.[4]

Extraction Techniques

As the *Emerald Tablet of Hermes Trismegistos* says, one must "separate the subtle from the gross, skillfully and with art." Oils must be separated from the plant material in which they are found, and different plants require different methods. Most are based on the premise that essential oils do not mix with water, or that they do mix with oils (fats) and/or alcohol.

Distillation

The plant material goes into a container called the body, and then a head is attached that tapers into a tube. The material is boiled or suspended over steam. By cooling the tube coming from the head, the vapors condense and drop into a collecting flask. The oil separates from the water, usually floating on top, and can be collected.

Solvents

Usually solvents are used for delicate blossoms like jasmine and narcissus. They are sealed in tanks with a solvent such as benzene or petroleum ether, into which the oils and waxes dissolve. Then the solvent, which has a low boiling point,

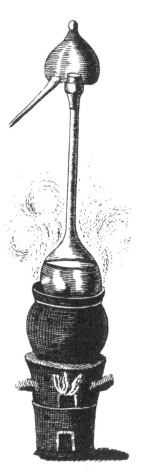

18th c. French glass still

is evaporated. Because of the presence of plant paraffins, a floral "concrete" results. Alcohol can then be used to make a tincture of the pure essence.

Enfleurage

This is one of the oldest techniques used by humans. The blossoms are carefully laid upon purified and refined lard, tallow, suet, or other similar—preferably aroma-free—material and enclosed to prevent the loss of their odors. When the flowers wilt in one or two days they are replaced with fresh flowers until the fat has reached the desired impregnation of fragrance. This pomade is then used directly or the essential oils are dissolved in alcohol.

Maceration

Similar to enfleurage, the plant material is first crushed, then soaked in oil or purified fat, strained, and more plant material added until the desired fragrance concentration is reached.

Expression

This method refers to the extraction of oils from the flesh, seeds, and skins of fruit by cold pressing. It is most often used with the skins of citrus fruit.

The Sense of Smell

Helen Keller, living with the absence of her visual sense, said, "smell is a potent wizard." In fact, the amount of our brain tissue devoted to smell is larger than that of our other senses, being tied to the limbic or old-brain system. The limbic system influences the entire endocrine system of hormones that regulates our bodily functions. Thus, smell can have a direct effect on any aspect of our lives, from the most basic things, like heartbeat and breathing, up to the most complex, like psychological stress and sexual arousal. In our noses, the olfactory nerves, or neurons—which conduct the messages about smells to the brain—are actually extensions of the brain. And unlike the neurons for our other senses, which are irreplaceable if damaged by disease or injury, the olfactory neurons constantly replicate themselves. This biological engineering is a strong indication of how important is the sense of smell, even if we don't normally consider it essential to our survival.

The sense of smell is our least understood sense. Natural body odors can determine who we are attracted to and who repulses us. Scents evoke memories and feelings, sympathies and antipathies, bypassing the conscious mind—which often has no clue as to the source of our reactions. Odors are keys that unlock our deepest memories. They affect our physical body via our hormones, heart rate, digestion, breathing, and immune system, to mention only a few. Some people with migraine headaches discover how intensely their sense of smell affects them, because their reactions to smell are greatly magnified at that time.

Exactly how smell works, and how we can distinguish among 10,000 different odors, is still one of the mysteries of the human body. Smell is inseparable from breathing and forms a major part of what we call "taste," which has only four perceptions of its own: salt, sour, sweet, and bitter—which can be extremely limiting, as people who have lost their sense of smell soon discover. The olfactory sense is the most powerful site of food recognition and protects us from foods that have gone bad.

High in the nose is the olfactory epithelium, two yellow-brown, mucus-covered smell receptors about the size of dimes, each consisting of about five million cells. Mucus in the nose keeps the receptors wet, because moisture heightens the sense of smell. A wet nose is a good nose. The receptors pick up volatile and lipid-soluble molecules using tiny filaments called cilia—about one thousand hairs per olfactory cell—which may be able to identify odor molecules by their shape and then stimulate the olfactory nerves.

It is currently believed that these odor receptors are coded by a huge family of genes to sense particular components of smell and produce a characteristic "fingerprint" pattern of activity in the brain.[5] As we shall see later, this fingerprint is surprisingly not that of the smell itself but an individualized composite based on the associations we have made to that smell in the past. On the whole, much of human response to olfaction seems to be learned. From the olfactory mucus membrane, signals are sent to "olfactory bulbs" that extend forward like tiny spoons from the brain. Odors are processed, and an electrical impulse travels along nerves, bypassing the neocortex or thinking brain, directly to the limbic system, part of the primitive or "old" brain, where they generate a reaction that is more emotional than mental. (Hearing and vision, in contrast, first stimulate the thalamus, which registers only warmth and pain.)

Damage to the limbus has been found to affect memory and cause eating disorders and sexual dysfunction. The "old" brain is directly connected to the hypothalamus and pituitary glands, and therefore to our immune system and hormones, but it also influences other kinds of thinking and creative processes. Author Diane Ackerman poetically describes it as "a mysterious, ancient, and intensely emotional section of our brain in which we feel, lust, and invent."[6] Smell was our first sense, and our brains actually grew from the olfactory stalks. Therefore, as Ackerman points out: "We think because we smell."[7]

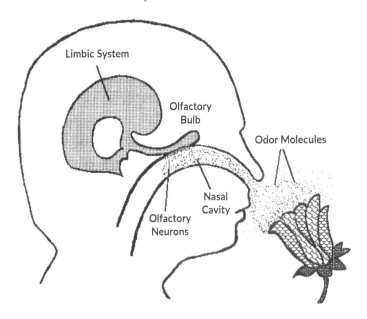

Smells affect our emotions most of all and can therefore be used to intentionally alter our state of consciousness. Smell memories are long term, sharp, and intense. In experiments, when a scent is present during learning, and then presented again during testing, recall is lower for those who did not have the accompanying scent.

It is difficult to be unhappy in a rose garden. Realtors know that it is hard to resist the allure of a home where bread or chocolate-chip cookies are baking. Tangerines bring out a sense of lighthearted play. Peppermint or lily of the valley helps keeps one alert. The aroma of vanilla is that of emotional nurturance mixed with sensuality; it helps one to relax. "New car" is a scent that makes us feel prosperous (and it can now be bought as an aerosol). The wearing of, and bathing with, perfumes has been indulged in every culture, especially for its known effect on sexual response—both psychological and physical.

An organ that detects pheromones (odors that trigger sexual behavior) called the "vomero-nasal organ" (VNO), previously found only in insects and animals, was finally discovered in human beings in October 1991. The word pheromone comes from the Greek *pherein*, meaning "to bear along," and *hormon*, "an excitement." It stimulates sexual response and can be detected in amounts as small as three-trillionths of an ounce.

In general, odor perception is most acute in childhood, falls off at about age eleven and again at eighteen. But some odors, like those similar to testosterone, are not perceived at all prior to puberty and are strongest to ovulating women (up to a thousand times stronger than at other times of the month). In fact, ovulating women themselves tend to smell "sweeter" to men. It is clear that hormones influence our sense of smell, but our sense of smell also influences our hormones. Girls who are never around men tend to have a late menarche. Similarly, a reduced sense of smell sharply reduces one's ability to respond sexually, and for women can create irregular menstrual periods.

Some oils like pine and cedar will cover disagreeable odors, so have been used in cleaning preparations. Irritating smells are used, such as that added to natural gas, to make it detectable in case of leaks. The smell of violets,

10   *Essence of Tarot*

on the other hand, slightly anesthetizes the nose, so that its odor seems to disappear quickly. Fragrances, both natural and chemical, are now routinely added to thousands of products, including soaps, diapers, dolls, insecticides, toilet paper, tampons, clothes hangers, garbage bags, candles, and cat litter. Manufacturers have learned that the public will tend to buy a scented product in preference to one that has no smell. A recent trend that significantly affects sales in fields as diverse as shoes, mobile phones, and computing devices is known as "scent marketing." A single brand may require the addition of millions of pounds of fragrance each year, and the use of fragrances continues to grow.

The Sociopolitics of Essence

There are few things that you can work with on a daily basis that come from as many different places in the world as essential oils: rose from Bulgaria, hyssop from Egypt, cardamom from Sri Lanka, frankincense from Somalia, lemongrass from Madagascar, nutmeg from Indonesia, patchouli from China, petitgrain from Paraguay, bois de rose (rosewood) from Brazil, angelica from Germany, pine from Siberia, vetiver from Haiti, ylang-ylang from the Philippines, jasmine from Morocco, sandalwood from India, spikenard from the Himalayas, tea tree and eucalyptus from Australia, orange and peppermint from the United States.

Yet along with the romance of evocative names and far-away places, we should recognize and take responsibility, where possible, for the social, economic, and political realities that underlie the world production of essential oils. Many fragrant plant materials are supplied by third-world countries, not only because they are exotic or indigenous but also because harvesting is labor-intensive, and there is an abundance of cheap labor available in poor and underdeveloped countries. Traditionally, this has led to the colonization and exploitation of other cultures and sometimes of women within those cultures. For example, in some parts of the world, women are barred from

Essential Oils

planting and harvesting work because of menstrual taboos, giving them no direct access to the cash economy. All external buying power, and thus political power, then rests in the hands of males.

Rich and privileged people have always used fragrances cosmetically and in their environment, while the poor would partake of fragrances only during rituals. Historically, conspicuous and frivolous consumption of oils and resins, worth far more than their weight in gold, were regularly burned, poured, and eaten during the parties and celebrations of the wealthy.

Animal rights and species endangerment are other pertinent issues. Some substances used in making fragrances come from animals slaughtered to obtain their secretions. Most are genitalia that are part of the animal's sexual allure. Musk (from the gut of an East Indian deer), especially, has a chemical component similar to testosterone and can cause women to ovulate more often and conceive more easily. Civet comes from an Ethiopian cat, and castoreum comes from Canadian and Russian beavers. In concentration, these are often foul-smelling but become quite sweet and pleasing when sufficiently diluted. Synthetic versions of these should be used in fragrances and not used at all in aromatherapy.

Environmental abuse is also of concern, and some plants and trees are being endangered by our increased demand for essential oils. Rosewood, for example, is being sacrificed daily in the Amazon rain forests and is not being replaced. In the United States, our native birches were nearly all cut in the 19th century for the oil called wintergreen.

The vagaries of weather—droughts, hurricanes, and the effects of global warming, for example—also play a part in the production, availability, and prices of essential oils.

As a consumer and user of essential oils, you should appreciate them not only for their intrinsic qualities but also for the human effort and societal and planetary costs involved in their production and distribution.

All organic life on earth depends on the symbiotic relationship between plants and animals—especially humans, who are the most numerous of the animals. For every breath we take, we use oxygen that is produced (exhaled) by plants, while we produce (exhale) the carbon dioxide they need to live. Plants are our beloved partners in the dance of life—it is not only their oils that are essential.

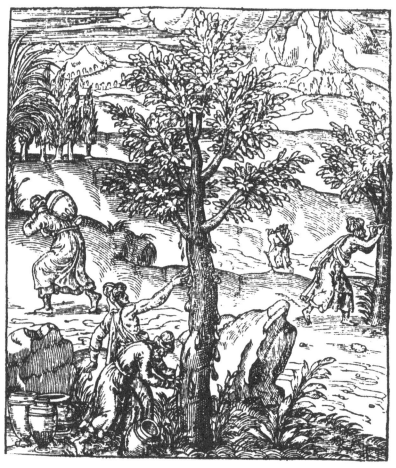

Collecting resins for incense. From *Cosmographie Universelle*, by Andre Thevet, 1575.

CHAPTER 2

A Magical History of Oils

*"Thou perceivest the Flowers put forth their precious Odours!
And none can tell how from so small a center comes such sweets
Forgetting that within the Center[,] Eternity expands
Its ever [en]during doors. . . ."*
—William Blake, *Milton*

Earliest Uses

Anthropologist Louis Leakey speculated that the earliest humans survived because predatory animals were repelled by their scent. In cultures where people relied on their senses for survival, they developed a sense of smell keen enough to track animals and may have used the oils from aromatic leaves to disguise their own scent. D. M. Stoddart postulates that monogamy was the direct result of the genetic selection of women, who, as plant gatherers, had their ovulatory scent signals masked by resins and oils and thus would mate only with bonded males. This also led, he believes, to the receptivity of females throughout their cycles.[1]

The earliest use of essential oils in magical rituals was as incense burned to attract the gods and keep evil spirits at bay and for ceremonial purification.

Leaves, twigs, and needles were ritually thrown into the fire as sacred offerings. Participants in such sacred rites entered into a mystical reverie conducive to contact with Spirit and discovered that they could revive that same state whenever they smelled the sacred plant offerings. Inhaling the smoke of certain plants induced trances, and words spoken while in this state were considered messages from the gods. Souls of the dead were believed to ascend to heaven with the smoke burned at their burial rites or from incense placed on bodies that were cremated.

Oils used in rites of initiation and consecration marked a person with a new odor and thus as of a new order. Spiritual persons and martyrs often smell sweet after death. This has been called the "Odor of Sanctity." For example, it is well documented that Swami Yogananda's body sweetly smelled of roses a week after his death. This effect was guaranteed to royalty and priests, who could afford rare incenses and oils.

Oils were also used for anointing, mummification and preservation of flesh, and in cosmetics. Cosmetics were originally magical, used as facial markings or masks that imitated the beneficial forces the wearer wished to contact or assume or to confuse the evil forces they wished to avoid. Kohl, used on the eyes, additionally served to shield them from the sun. Priestesses and priests were the earliest perfumers, just as they were also the healers, and the same plants were used for both. One way to recognize a possible medicinal herb is by a strong smell indicating the presence of essential oils. Shamans had special olfactory powers, using smell to recognize not only possible healing plants but also disease, weakness, and fear. Sometimes epileptics were shamans because of their amazing ability to be seized from this world and transported into another—and then return. Seizures are often preceded by odor hallucinations (phantosmia) and can be triggered by certain odors. Around the world, perfumes came to be associated with a kind of love-magic that bewitches and entrances its victims. As cities came into being, oils and incenses were used more and more by the privileged to exorcise the disagreeable smells of urban living conditions.

The following short sections on the historical use of incenses and fragrances in magic and rituals are intended to present interesting examples of how people from around the world have used aromatics. Since you may wish to adapt some of these when creating your own rituals, note which ones especially appeal to you.

Babylon and Mesopotamia

In Mesopotamia it was believed that the dead lived upon the smoke of incense burned by their descendants. Their word for incense, *ntyw*, appears among their earliest written texts, and was probably an aromatic wood. Babylonian priests ceremonially opened the mouths and eyes of statues of the gods and goddesses each morning by using a compound of myrrh and olive oil. According to Magical Magpie (a collector of perfume lore), "the oldest known incense formula comes from Babylon where rock rose, myrrh, honey and storax in equal amounts were burned to the gods at the New Year's celebration. He gives Astarte's traditional incense as a combination of myrrh, musk, rose, and jasmine.[2] The ancient Akkadian word for Lebanon, *lebanatu*, means "incense," as the country was named after its famed cedars, which were a major source of aromatic woods and oils.

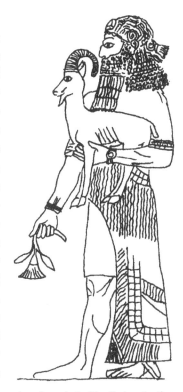

Assyrian priest with offerings for the gods: a goat and a fragrant flower.

In Assyria, according to Strabo, incense was always offered to the goddess of love and fertility immediately after sexual intercourse.

A Magical History of Oils

Egypt

Queen Hatshepsut (circa 1500 BCE) was famed for her early explorations and trade with the lands of Punt. These are the earliest references to frankincense and myrrh. Burial sites are often filled with ointment jars and aromatic flagons, many of which still retain their odor after thousands of years. Cleopatra (69–30 BCE) experimented with fragrances and was known as a sorceress and an alchemist. She covered the sails of her boat with scented oils so that—as she sailed down the Nile, the people would know that a goddess was passing. Mark Anthony, to please her, gave her a nine-room perfume and cosmetic factory on the Dead Sea near the En Gedi oasis.

Anubis, the dog-headed deity who guarded the gates of the underworld, checked each man for his odor. In a passage from the Book of the Dead, Anubis announces to the initiates of the mysteries that he hears "the voice of a man who cometh from the land of desire, he is one who knoweth our path and our dwelling place, and I am satisfied for I smell his odour as one of yourselves."[3]

The Egyptians believed there were several nonphysical aspects to each human being. The *Khaibt,* represented hieroglyphically by an open fan, implied the odor or aura of a person and included the sympathetic or antipathetic influence of one being on another.[4]

Ancient Egypt's favorite scent, called *Kyphi,* was used both internally as medicine and externally as odorant. One traditional recipe contained myrrh, calamus (sweet flag), juniper, and coriander, while another adds to this cypress, henna flowers (camphire), and mint mixed in honey.[5] Woods, resins, blossoms, and oils were used for fumigations, embalming, and incense to exorcise the demons of disease from the body of a sick person. The primary ingredients in mummification were myrrh, oakmoss, and pine resin (which are highly antibiotic and antimicrobial). The body cavity was filled with myrrh mixed with cassia blossoms. Essential oils and resins exceeded the value of precious metals and gems, as demonstrated by the fact that King

Tut's tomb, for instance, held more than one hundred gallons of scented oils and emollients. Grave robbers took the oils but left the containers and most other objects of value behind.

Egyptian paintings and reliefs show women with small cones atop their heads. These were scented fats and aromatics that melted with the heat of the day, coating the hair and body with protective cremes and releasing a pleasing fragrance. The fats were usually from animals, including the lion, hippopotamus, snake, crocodile, cat, and ibex. The 19th-century English magician MacGregor Mathers explained that the cones additionally symbolized the flame of the divine spirit. "The whole idea of the dress of the priestess is that the life of matter is purified and ruled by the divine spirit of life from above."[6]

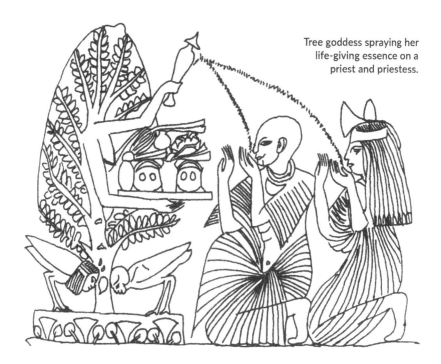

Tree goddess spraying her life-giving essence on a priest and priestess.

A Magical History of Oils

Priests bathed thrice daily, followed by an application of oils and unguents. Another unique item was the perfume spoon—long, narrow, and almost flat—on which odorous substances could be carried and burned.

The paramount fragrant plant of the Egyptians was the blue water lily (lotus) or *Nymphaea nouchali var. coerulea*. The bright yellow center viewed against the blue petals represented the sun god Ra crossing the sky, and signified the resurrection of Osiris. As it contains several narcotic and hallucinogenic substances, its use in wine and ointments must have produced interesting effects. Other popular scents included the night-blooming white waterlily and henna flowers (camphire), as well as the "Balm of Gilead."

The finest olive oil was made from unripe olives and was very dark and viscous. Balanos oil came from the kernels of a tree (*Balanites aegiptiaca*) whose leaves contained unusual markings. Thus it was said that Thoth, god of wisdom and magic, inscribed the names of priests and pharaohs on the leaves. Different incense mixtures were offered at different times of the day; for instance, as the sun would set, Ra would be offered a special blend—usually Kyphi—to strengthen him for his journey through darkness.

Hebrews

The Tree of Life in the garden of Eden, from which ran four rivers, may itself have been an odoriferous tree and the rivers its fragrant sap. One river is specifically stated to have contained bdellium (*Commiphora erythraea*), a gum resin used in incense, perfumes, and medicines.

The Jews did not begin using incense in quantity until after their return from captivity in Egypt around 1200 BCE, when they conquered the Canaanites (Phoenicians), one of whose gods was called Baal Hamon ("Lord of the Perfumed Altar"). Two types were used: one consisted entirely of frankincense, and the other a compound of frankincense with various aromatic spices—stacte, onycha, and galbanum. Only priests were permitted to offer these incenses as a sacrifice on the altar. The Bible relates a story of King

Uzziah who arrogantly presumed to offer incense in the Temple and was punished with leprosy (II Chronicles 26:16,19).

The oil used for anointing the altar, and all altar objects, and for consecrating high priests included: 500 shekels each of myrrh and cassia and 250 shekels each of cinnamon and sweet calamus in olive oil, while another version adds frankincense and labdanum (rock rose). Moses sent his brother Aaron with fumigating incense to protect his people from a plague that was ravaging the land (Numbers 17:11–15). Myrtle (*hadas*), sacred to Astarte and Aphrodite, was also associated with Queen Esther whose Hebrew name was *Hadassah* ("myrtle tree"). She spent a year being bathed in special oils before her marriage.

Isaiah describes the daughters of Zion as owning "soul boxes," "houses of the soul," or "perfume boxes" as they have been variously translated. According to biblical scholar Theodor Gaster, these were containers of fragrance that acted as

amulets in which the soul of the wearer was supposed to lodge . . . for in the eyes of a people who, like the Hebrews, identified the principle of life with the breath, the mere act of smelling a perfume might easily assume a spiritual aspect; the scented breath inhaled might seem an accession of life, an addition made to the essence of the soul. Hence it would be natural to regard the fragrant object itself . . . as a centre of radiant spiritual energy, and therefore as a fitting place into which to breathe out the soul whenever it was deemed desirable to do so for a time.[7]

In the *Song of Solomon*, the Queen of Sheba describes her love for Solomon in terms of fragrances of great worth.

While the king was at his repose,
my spikenard sent forth the odor thereof.
A bundle of myrrh is my beloved unto me;
he shall lay all night between my breasts.
My beloved is unto me as a cluster of camphire[8]
in the vineyards of En Gedi.[9]

Frankincense, signifying divinity, and myrrh, meaning "bitter" and therefore signifying persecution and death, were brought to Jesus at birth by the three Magi or magicians, thus foretelling his purpose in incarnation. Myrrh was also used to prepare his body for burial (John 19:39), and myrrh in wine was offered to Jesus at the crucifixion, possibly as an analgesic in addition to its deeper symbolism.

The term "Christos" means "the anointed one," and Jesus was anointed by Mary Magdalene, a temple priestess of the goddess Astarte, in the ritual of Chrism (Mark 14:3, John 12:3). In Bethany, at the house of Simon the leper, Magdalene used an ointment of spikenard (a valerian plant from the Himalayan mountains, *Nardostachys jatamansi*)—which filled the house with its mossy, earthy odor—to anoint the feet of Jesus and wipe them with her hair. Aromatherapist Victoria Edwards, who has extensively researched spikenard and the legends of Mary Magdalene, explains that "the ancient ritual of Chrism is referred to in the Nag Hammadi Library as more important than baptism and reaches even farther back to King Malchezedeck who first introduced the ritual of bread and wine and oil."[10]

Maria Prophetissa, known as Mary the Jewess (1st to 3rd centuries CE), was described by Zosimos of Panopolis (Graeco-Egyptian alchemist) as Miriam, the sister of Moses. According to alchemical legend, she invented Western distillation using her alchemical apparatus called the *Kerotakis.* She is reputedly the inventor of the "water-bath" (double-boiler), still called the "bain-marie" in France. She is also remembered for her explication of unity in diversity: "One becomes two, two becomes three, and out of the third comes the one as the fourth." She spoke eloquently of marrying the white and red gums (probably odorous resins) as a symbol of the alchemical *conjunctio* or mystic marriage and described alchemical water (essential oil separated through distillation) as an angel who descends from the sky.[11]

Greeks and Romans

The Greeks ascribed a divine origin to all aromatic plants. Chloris, "the Green One," was the Greek goddess of flowers, as Flora was the Roman. Their rites of new life, celebrated at the beginning of May, were, as author Barbara Walker points out, "attended by sexual license and lascivious behavior."[12] Their mystic energy was the secret of all life. Dionysus was god of the scents and flavors of wines and perfumes. Aphrodite was the first user of aromatics, but this knowledge was stolen by her nymph, the prophetess Ænone, who gave it to her husband Paris. Naughty Paris then told Helen of Troy, thus guaranteeing her the unsurpassed beauty that caused the Trojan War. The Bacchanals ate poisonous ivy, which perhaps caused their mad dancing on the hillsides. The priestesses at Delphi were anointed with hallucinogenic oils, or leaned over brasiers of burning bay (laurel) leaves in order to discover the oracles for which they became famous. The priestess of the oracle at Patras would pray and offer incense; then, gazing into a mirror or a sacred well, would seek an answer. According to Homer, the powerful sorceress Circe kept Odysseus on her island with the seductive fragrance of essential oils. Homer described the great goddess Hera as bathed in fragrance:

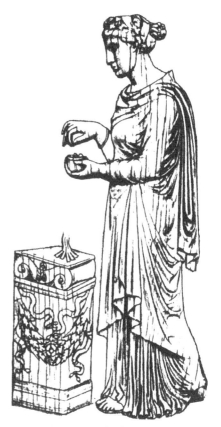

Priestess offering incense on an altar; Rome, c. 400 CE

A Magical History of Oils

Her feet she bathes and round her body pours
Soft oil of fragrances and ambrosial showers.
The winds perfumed the balmy gale conveys
Through heaven, through earth and all the aerial ways.[13]

In Greece, each part of the body was anointed with a different oil: mint for the arms, palm oil for the jaws and breast, marjoram for eyebrows and hair, and ground ivy or thyme for the knees and neck. Ground ivy was said to keep the mind clear. Pythagoras advocated that the gods be worshipped with incense rather than animal sacrifices and thus changed the practice of sacrifice.

In Rome, incense came to be used for the victory marches of returning generals. Every Greek and Roman household eventually had an altar on which incense was burned, and at dinner parties the sense of smell was stimulated as much as the sense of taste, both in air and food. Perfume manufacturers were called *unguentarii*, from whence we get the term "unguent."

India

In 1975, Dr. Paolo Rovesti, investigating the Indus Valley civilization, discovered a perfectly preserved distillation apparatus made of terracotta from 3000 BCE, accompanied by perfume containers.[14] Previously it was believed that distillation was first discovered by the Arabs in about 1000 CE—4,000 years later! India developed fine flower oils and discovered the use of sandalwood, not only to induce calm but also to repel termites. Sandalwood was therefore used for both its mystical properties as an oil and as lumber from which to construct temples and sacred images that were impervious to pests. Hindu sibyls called *dainyals* used cloths over their heads (like their sisters in Greece, Africa, Java, and South America) to inhale smoke—in this case from the sacred cedar—until seized by convulsions, after which they would sing prophetic chants. Each deity in the Hindu pantheon had its own favored fragrance. And perfumed waters were offered for washing the body of the gods. In marriage celebrations, flowers were strewn on the bed to relax the bride and surround her with beauty.

The sexual/mystical/spiritual system of Tantra, which originated in India well over 1,000 years ago, uses fragrances extensively in love rituals, as this passage from *Sexual Secrets* indicates:

> Before sexual union, the female partner is worshipped as the embodiment of the creative force, the Shakti or Wisdom-energy; her body parts are then anointed with different perfumes to honor her creative role and lift up her psyche so she can truly manifest as a goddess. In the sexual rite known as the Rite of the Five Essentials . . . the finest oil of jasmine is applied to the hands, oil of patchouli or keora to the neck and cheeks, essence of amber or hina musk to the breasts, extract of spikenard or valerian to the hair, musk from the musk deer to the sexual region, oil of sandalwood to the thighs and essence of saffron to the feet of the woman. For the male partner, sandalwood oil or paste is applied to the forehead, neck, chest, navel, sexual region, upper arms, thighs, hands and feet.[15]

In Ayurveda, incense is used as a method of balancing *doshas*. Scents derived from natural ingredients are believed to exert healing powers upon body, mind, and spirit. Ayurveda organizes plant parts elementally, which enables one to create individualized balancing prescriptions. For example, roots used in perfumery—such as turmeric, ginger, and spikenard—are classified as belonging to the element of earth, while branches and stems—such as aloes, cassia, frankincense, myrrh, and sandalwood—are classified as belonging to the water element. Leaves are air, while flowers are fire.

China

Joss sticks—in which aromatic compounds were bound to a stick with glue—were invented in China. Among the ten thousand rites of the Taoist sect, it is said that the "burning of incense has primacy."[16] Buddhist monks were branded during ordination ceremonies called "receiving the fire," in which a cone of incense burned down to their shaven foreheads.[17]

A Magical History of Oils

Documented evidence of incense in China dates back to the Neolithic era. By the Song dynasty, which began in 960 CE, incense in conjunction with Zen Buddhist philosophy became an intrinsic aspect of meditation. Items that have been identified as incense censers date back as far as the Warring States period, approximately 475 BCE to 221 BCE. Incense censers and stationary burners are often ingenious works of art; for example, burners crafted to resemble mountain peaks with emanating plumes of incense smoke appearing to form clouds around them.

China was the terminus point for the Silk Road and so for centuries was able to sell and receive rare plants and other fragrance materials, including sandalwood from India and benzoin from Persia. Agarwood, also known as aloes or oudh (*Aquilaria* spp.), is a component in most traditional Chinese blends, although rarely if ever used alone, as it is perceived as being aggressively yang.

Fragrance played a significant role in China's varied spiritual traditions. Confucius was a great admirer of orchids, many of which have strong and distinctive aromas, while in traditional Taoist belief, extracting a plant's fragrance—for example, to create perfume or incense—is perceived as akin to liberating its soul.

Japan

In Japan, incense—first mentioned in 595 CE—was deliberately used to enhance appreciation of the four seasons, and both the Chinese and Japanese cultivated their ability to "listen to" rather than "smell" incense as a poetic accomplishment. In Japan, "listening to incense" was formalized into a ceremony called Koh-do, complementing the tea ceremony.[18] By the 16th century, ten virtues of Koh (incense) were recognized. Incense was said to bring communication with the transcendent, purify mind and body, remove uncleanliness, keep you alert, be a companion in the midst of solitude, and bring a moment of peace amidst busy affairs. Even when plentiful, one never tires of it; age does not change its efficacy; and, finally, used every day, it does no harm.[19]

The spirits of those who have sold bad incense, called Jiki Ko Ki, are punished by having to eat only the smoke of burning incense for all eternity. The Japanese equivalent of the Indian Devatas, called the Tennyo, are heavenly musicians who fill the air with flowers and perfumes. To pious Buddhists, they are ministering angels, but they sometimes assume the shape of women to make love to men.[20]

Mexico, Central and South America

They generally use tree resins and aromatic balsams as an incense. The most famous example would be copal, a resin deriving from *Protium copal* or the copal tree, which is indigenous to Mexico and Central America. Copal was used as incense prior to the arrival of the conquistadors. Its name derives from *copalli*, a Nahuatl word used to describe aromatic smoke or incense. (Nahuatl is the language of the Aztecs.) Copal was counted among the acceptable tributes delivered to the ruling Aztecs by those peoples whom they had conquered. It is believed to enhance divination.

Because the Aztecs had used copal in their own sacred ceremonies, it was forbidden for use as church incense by the conquering Spaniards, who imported frankincense from Europe instead. It wasn't until the late 19th century that copal and other indigenous incenses were permitted for use in Roman Catholic rites. Copal is believed to ward off malefic spirits, provide protection, and promote good health.

Copal remains an integral component of modern Day of the Dead (*Dias de los Muertos*) rituals, as does the scent of *cempasuchil*, or the Aztec marigold (*Tagetes erecta*). The scent of *cempasuchil* beckons the ancestors and other dead souls. Paths are created from the fresh flowers to lead the dead on their proper paths.

Tagetes lucida, another Mexican marigold, known as *yauhtli* or the sweet-scented marigold, possesses psychoactive properties and was used as an incense before the Spanish conquest. It is considered a profound ritual plant by the Huichols, an indigenous people of Mexico's Sierra Madre mountains.

A Magical History of Oils

Now widely touted as the "world's most popular fragrance," vanilla (*Vanilla planifolia*) derives from a species of orchid native to Mexico. It has been used ritually and therapeutically, as well as in perfumery and cosmetics. Vanilla bears a reputation—ancient and modern—as an aphrodisiac. The word "orchid" derives from a Greek word that literally means "testicle," while "vanilla," the name given the plant by the Spanish conquistadors, ultimately derives from a Latin word that can be translated as "little vagina." (The Aztecs called it *tlilxochitl*, meaning "black flower.") Vanilla was sacred to the Totonac, an indigenous people of Mexico, who incorporated it into ritual offerings. When the Aztecs conquered them in the mid-15th century, they incorporated vanilla into *xocalotl*, the Aztec hot chocolate drink. Meanwhile, the Mayans combined vanilla with copal in order to create temple incense.

The name of Balsam of Peru or Peru Balsam (*Myrosperum pereira*) is a misnomer. This fragrant resin derives from a Central American tree, primarily found in what is now El Salvador. However, Spanish conquerors transported the resin to Peru from whence it was shipped to Europe. Recipients assumed that Peru was its origin.

Palo Santo (*Bursera graveolens*) derives from a tree that is native mainly to Ecuador, Peru, and the Yucatán Peninsula in Mexico. Its name literally means "sacred wood" or "holy wood." Only wood that has naturally fallen from the tree may be used to make the incense, not only to preserve the living trees but also because both the fragrance and the tree spirit inside increases in potency after several years on the forest floor. Palo Santo has deep ties to shamanic rituals and is used in purification rites. It is burned as incense and also made into an essential oil.

Indigenous North Americans

The Inuit believed that the soul comes and goes through the nose. Fragrant botanicals have long held sacred significance throughout indigenous North America. Native American people have generally used cedar, pinon, sweet grass, and sage brush as incense, as fumigants, and for purification in sweat lodges. Different Native nations incorporate different plants into their sweat lodge rituals. For example, cedar and sage may be spread on the sweat lodge floor, while juniper leaves may be thrown on the lodge's heated stones.

Osha, or bear root (*Ligusticum porteri*), is among the most significant sacred plants of North America. It has been used for sacred, therapeutic, and talismanic purposes. Osha's fragrance is reputed to provide purification, as well as protection against malefic magic. In his book, *Plants of Power: Native American Ceremony and the Use of Sacred Plants* (Native Voices, 2002), Alfred Savinelli writes that "The Klamath Falls women burn osha root, using the smoke to perfume their hair and clothing." Osha should only be obtained from reputable sources, as it bears a strong resemblance to poison hemlock and water hemlock and is easily confused with these highly poisonous plants.

Herb bundles are traditionally crafted by tying dried herbs together to form a fragrant botanical wand. When these are burned, the smoke is wafted around the area to provide cleansing, protection, and purification. Although various botanicals are traditionally used, the most famous is white sage (*Salvia apiana*), which is native to the southwestern US, as well as coastal southern California and Mexico's Baja California peninsula. In the 21st century, white sage has become virtually synonymous with purification rituals, leading to charges of appropriation. Its popularity in mainstream culture has led to habitat loss, while its price has become prohibitive for indigenous users. Plant poachers wildcraft white sage in ways that are harmful and endanger the plants in order to sell them for mass production of herb bundles or "smudge sticks." It is recommended that those who wish to use white sage grow their own or purchase only from reputable growers.

Sweetgrass (*Hierochloe odorata*), also called holy grass, is an aromatic herb that grows at northern latitudes in what is now the US and Canada but also in Poland and Russia, where it is known as bison grass or buffalo grass. The plant is hardy enough to grow within the Arctic Circle. Sweetgrass has many uses, including spiritual, medicinal, cosmetic, and as a flavoring agent. Among the Haudenosaunee or Iroquois, sweetgrass has traditionally been used as an incense and as perfume.

Sweetgrass beckons benevolent spirits but is distasteful to malefic spirits. Among the most significant sacred herbs of Indigenous America, it is burned as incense. Sweetgrass braids are traditional spiritual offerings. Among many Native nations, including the Cree and the Ojibwe, sweetgrass is considered the eldest of all plants and is widely understood to be the hair of Mother Earth.

Europe

The Crusaders returned to Europe from the East with Oriental perfumes, causing the priesthood to declare that scent was associated with satanism. The Book of Enoch declared that fallen angels came to women and "taught them charms and enchantments, and made them acquainted with the cutting of roots and woods." Yet despite periodic objections, incense continued its use through the Eastern and Roman Catholic as well as Anglican Churches. This was the beginning of the vastly lucrative "spice" trade, in which "spice" was the general name for all aromatics. Rosaries, used by Catholics to count prayers to the Virgin Mary, were originally made out of beads of cooked and pressed rose petals that released their heavenly fragrance when fingered. In the 12th century, the Benedictine abbess and mystic Hildegard of Bingen was known for her distillation of lavender water. Marco Polo went to the Orient in the 13th century to obtain spices, and the great explorations of the 15th century, during which America was "discovered," were in search of better trade routes to the spice lands. The first alcohol-based perfume was not made until 1370. Known as Hungary Water and based on the oils of rosemary and lavender, its invention was attributed to Queen Elizabeth of Hungary.

King George III of England (1738–1820) declared the use of scents to seduce or betray someone into matrimony to be witchcraft—no doubt because of its widespread and effective application. Witches were thought to be able to fly after being anointed with certain plant oils, although modern commentators think it more likely that the hallucinogenic qualities of the ingredients enabled the witches to leave their bodies and fly astrally. Nevertheless, a 19th-century Anglican prayer recounts a medieval tale of the three Maries who brought the spices of virtuous works and prayers to the angel who stood before the tomb of Christ. The prayer concludes by asking that we may be filled by the hands of angels, like a censer, with the spice of God's blessing in order to send up pleasing prayers.

> "O God, to whose sepulchre . . . there came in the early morning women with spices, like holy souls carrying the virtues of holy works; and in whose sight there stood an angel, having a golden censer, . . . to whom incense was given to add to the prayers of all the saints before the throne of the Lord. . . . Fill this censer with thy heavenly blessing, that whosoever may perceive the fragrance of incense from it, may by the gift of thy boundless mercy send up the savours of holy prayers before the sight of thy majesty, by the hands of holy angels; through Jesus Christ."

Arabia and Islam

Ibn Sina Avicenna (980–1037 CE), an Arabic philosopher and physician, is reputed to have discovered the process of preserving scents by alcohol distillation and, in effect, invented perfume.

The Arabs have many beautiful legends about the origins of plants that are attributed to Muhammad. For example, it is said that the geranium first blossomed from a common hedge when Muhammad hung his washed shirt there to dry. And the first rose sprang up from the place where his sweat fell to the earth: "Whoever would smell my scent, let him smell the rose." Myrtle was also highly esteemed in Muslim lore. When Adam and Eve fell from paradise, they brought with them three things: the myrtle (chief of sweet-smelling flowers), wheat (chief of foods), and dates (chief of fruits). Muhammad is also reputed to have said, "There are three things of this world that I have been made to prefer: prayer, women, and scents."

A Magical History of Oils

To Arabs, it is thought that to deny someone your breath while talking is an insult, and therefore they stand closer to each other than is typical in the West. This may not be so strange, because a person's health and emotions (and their diet) can be perceived through their odor, so this is an act of honesty and affinity. Arabs also wash their noses with water each morning to expel demons that may enter the body at night through the nose.

The Sufi dervishes at one time held a monopoly on making scented unguents and cosmetics, and scents were employed in Arabic universities to stimulate thinking and creativity.

Persia (Iran)

The Persians believed that the righteous, after death, gave forth a sweet odor, and the person approaching the blissful regions of paradise were surrounded by a perfumed breeze.

Perfume was considered emblematic of wealth for ancient Persians, who inherited many of the perfumery practices of the Mesopotamians. Fragrances were used in spiritual rituals but also used to create fragrantly scented personal spaces. The kings of Persia possessed personal perfume blends that were forbidden to all others. Some theorize that this is the origin of the concept of personal fragrance blends, such as those created by modern perfumers today.

Fine fragrances and infused waters were produced during the Sassanian era (224 CE–651 CE). Archaeologists have discovered equipment and apparatuses for creating rosewater in ancient Kashan, where a rosewater festival is still held annually in modern Iran. The Sassanians practiced Zoroastrianism, an indigenous religion of Persia. Zoroastrian worship and ceremonies are held in sacred fire temples. Fire represents divine light for Zoroastrians and is intrinsic to the religion along with an ancient incense heritage. Plants used as incense in Zoroastrian fire rituals include agarwood and sandalwood. Zoroastrian sacred texts, including the Avesta, mention aromatics and incense.

Alchemy

Diane Ackerman points out in her book *A Natural History of the Senses* that we "cook" (transform) the air we breathe. "There is a furnace in our cells, and when we breathe we pass the world through our bodies, brew it lightly, and turn it loose again, gently altered for having known us."[21] As we shall see, this is the most subtle form of physical alchemy.

Alchemy has a long history that I will not attempt to recap here. Most of us have heard of the search for the Philosopher's Stone to transmute lead into gold, but a second type of alchemy consisted of the search for the Elixir of Life. This was a botanical essence of great power and was represented on the earthly plane by lengthily and delicately prepared tinctures, waters, spiritualized homeopathic salts, unguents, oils, and perfumes.

Alchemy works simultaneously on the physical and spiritual planes, for its premise is that a spark of the Divine exists in all matter and that we can discover it, both in physical objects and in ourselves. As the 19th-century magician W. Wynn Westcott said, "The Higher Alchymy then is almost identical with Religion. . . . The function of Religion and the Great Work of the Alchymist is Spiritualization. The separation of the subtle from the gross; the redemption of spirit, while still *seated* in matter, from the taint inevitable to the lowest planes of manifestation."[22] In alchemy, both spirit and matter constantly reflect each other, "as above, so below."

All acts in alchemy are metaphor. The alchemist's furnace comes from the baker's oven, which itself represents the womb and suggests the place of transformation from seed into the staff of life. The transmutation of base matter into gold—the central image of alchemy—is itself a metaphor for its real objective, which is the transmutation of the alchemist from the base matter of flesh into the pure gold of the spirit. Just as one learns natural law from dealing with botany and chemistry and coming to understand their transformations—in which all impurities are refined, burned, calcinated, and evaporated away—so the alchemist, by a conscious effort on the spiritual plane, discovers the methods of self-transmutation.

A Magical History of Oils

The method of alchemical transformation is given in the *Alchemist's Handbook* by 20th-century alchemist Frater Albertus: "Alchemy is the raising of the vibrations."[23] He continues: "Since everything that grows comes from a seed, the fruit must be contained in its seed. Mark this well, for here lies the secret of creation. . . . This is nothing else but transmutation."[24] We can help bring the products of creation to perfection but only in harmony with nature's laws. To discover the essence of nature, it is important to discover the essence of her plants.

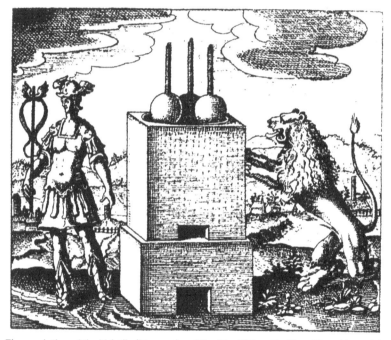

The resolution of the Volatile (Mercury) and the Fixed (Lion=Sun) is achieved in a triple operation in the alchemist's furnace. From *Philosophia reformata*, Frankfurt, 1622.

The aroma molecules of plants represent what is called the quintessence, and the original techniques for distillation of plant materials emerged from alchemical experiments to extract them in their purest state. In the *Emerald Tablet of Hermes*, it says: "Distilling is no other thing, but only a purifying of the gross from the subtle, and the subtle from the gross." In other words, the alchemist must "sublimate that which is bodily, and embody that which is spirit." This can be translated as the oils in the plant material ("bodily") were evaporated ("sublimate") and then condensed ("embody") into the odoriferous essence of the plant, whose ethereal molecules were themselves the quintessence.

Frater Albertus tells us "the life force is a separate essence which fills the universe. This essence, or fifth essence (quintessence), is the truly important object that alchemists seek. It is the most important one for the alchemist to find and then to separate."[25] Of course, most essential oils today are not prepared with anything like an alchemist's consciousness, but they can be used with the intention of raising the vibrations of whatever we are doing. Using them, we plant a seed of consciousness whose fruit is the sacred space that allows us to know the perfection of the universe. Francis Barrett in *The Magus* explains: "Because our spirit is pure subtle, lucid, airy and unctuous . . . nothing, therefore, is better adapted . . . than like vapours which are more suitable to our spirit in substance; for then, by reason of their likeness, they do more to stir up, attract and transform the spirit."[26]

Florence Farr, then Chief in Anglia of the Hermetic Order of the Golden Dawn, who studied and practiced Egyptian magic, explained in her commentary on a 1655 book on alchemy called *Euphrates of the Waters of the East* by Eugenius Philalethes:

> This odor or aura is especially noticeable in vegetable life. It is found that the essential oil existing in the outer cells of the petals is the source of the perfume of a flower, the lower surfaces containing tannin and coloring matter. Now the first action of the Foundation of life [Yesod on the Tree of Life] is to emit an odorous sphere or aura or emanation of influence. From the interaction of this with the Ruach or spirit, the material body is formulated from the elements. The seed being

A Magical History of Oils

the magnet of attraction I may here remark that after fermentation or putrefaction, an amount of a volatile oil far exceeding in quantity the original essential oil of a natural substance can be extracted from it by the usual processes of distillation, etc. . . . We may gather that the essential oil, and comprehend with it the perfume or aura, was the physical basis of life in the eyes of the ancients. Death, putrefaction or fermentation sets free large quantities of this essence which when treated by the wise, may effect (sic) the regeneration of a particular body. Bringing about by art in a short time what nature would have effected (sic) slowly.[27]

CHAPTER 3

About the Tarot

*"We cannot see the soul until we experience it,
and we cannot understand the dream until we enter it."*
—Dr. James Hillman, analyst and author

Basic Information

The tarot deck consists of seventy-eight cards divided into the Major and Minor Arcana. The twenty-two cards of the Major Arcana represent twenty-two lessons, archetypes, keys, paths, steps, angels, essences, or aspects of the individual. They embody the secret teachings of the ages—each one a messenger of the self to the Self.

The Minor Arcana consist of sixteen court cards and forty number, or pip, cards. They are divided into four suits corresponding to the four elements: Wands (fire), Cups (water), Swords (air), and Pentacles (earth). The four court cards (or what I call people cards) have many different attributions, ranging from Shaman, Priestess, Son, and Daughter to the traditional King, Queen, Knight, and Page. The number cards are the ace through 10 of each suit. In a reading, the people cards tell you *who else* in your life or what part of *yourself* is involved in the situation. The number cards describe *what*—what is the situation you are involved in, and the Major Arcana tell you *why*—why you are involved in this situation, and they often represent a need within yourself. If you are new to the tarot, spread all the cards out, in order, on the floor, and examine their sequencing and interrelationships.

You can use any deck you like, but my comments in this book are based primarily on the Rider-Waite-Smith tarot (and its many variations), the Harris-Crowley Thoth deck, the Major Arcana of the Marseilles deck, and the Motherpeace deck. I prefer decks that have pictures on all the cards, because they present varied visual and symbolic options for interpreting them. With these decks, you can respond directly to the images and not just to meanings you memorize or look up in a book.

MINOR ARCANA SUITS CHART		
Symbol	Suit—Element	Meaning of the Suits
	WANDS—Fire	Self-growth. Spirit. Inspiration. Energy. Creativity. Initiation. Enthusiasm. Desire. Passion. Perception. Action. Movement. Optimism.
	CUPS—Water	Feeling & Emotions. Unconscious. Imagination. Intuition. Being psychic. Dreams. Visualization. Inner Processes. Relationships. Receptivity. Reflection.
	SWORDS—Air	Thoughts. Struggles. Conflict. Decisions. Analysis. Wit & Cunning. Discussion. Communication. Mental Processes. Acuity. Criticism. Pessimism.
	PENTACLES—Earth	Results. Actualization. Sensation. Security. Tradition. Grounding. Centeredness. Manifestation. Skills. Craftsmanship. Rewards for Accomplishment. Fruits of Labor.

History

The history of the tarot is fairly recent, especially compared to aromatics. The tarot as we know it dates only from the mid-15th century, appearing first in northern Italy as a game. Nevertheless, it is possible that the images, especially those in the Major Arcana, were invented to record mysteries that had been passed primarily from mouth to ear for thousands of years. All other games that were based, at least in part, on "chance," were, in their original forms, attempts to allow the will of the Divine to be known to humans—and so too the tarot. I like to think that if tarot and scents had ever been linked in the past, it might have been in Egypt in the initiation chambers under the Sphinx and the Great Pyramid.

It is even possible to speculate that images used together with scents date back to as long ago as the amazing city of Mohenjo-Daro in the Indus Valley. It is there that the 5,000-year-old perfume distillery and containers were found; but, in addition, thousands of small clay tablets were dug up that had simple images of animals and other markings stamped upon them. There are two theories about these tablets, and I think both may be true: 1) that they were used in some kind of "game" (i.e., divination), and 2) that they were merchants' markers and therefore used in the spice trade. Mohenjo-Daro was at the center of the ancient world—linking Europe and Africa to Indo-China. Therefore, a tablet depicting a deer may have indicated the transport of musk, and in the game, it is fun to speculate that the same tablet may have stood for something like speed or virility or sexual appeal. The illustrated seal shows the sacred asratha tree from whose branches grow animal heads symbolizing fertility.

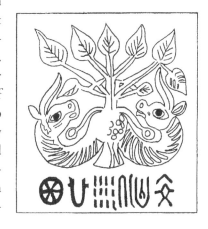

Aromatics and tarot are linked by their mutual associations with mystery, emotions, enchantment, and transformation. They both also partake of the unworldly and the ethereal, and each seems a gift of the Spirit, a link to the soul. Both have been called the work of the devil, because people have feared that hidden secrets might be revealed through their use. Psychotherapist Dr. J. Pratt noted in 1942 that perfumes "unconsciously reveal what consciously they aim to hide."[1]

The Rider-Waite-Smith tarot (RWS) does include several references to specific plants, and one deck, *The Herbal Tarot* created by Candice Cantin and

Michael Tierra, takes this even further to suggest a specific medicinal plant for each card.[2] This is based on the premise that by linking a plant with its most closely related tarot card, the knowledge and uses of each will be expanded. This premise also applies to linking essential oils with tarot cards. A long tradition—based on what is called the "law of correspondence"—for such an association has existed for centuries, being tested and modified continually up to the present day. You are invited here to be part of this experience.

The Law of Correspondence

Central to the doctrine of the "Ageless Wisdom," including magic and alchemy, is what is called the law of correspondence. This law states that everything in the universe is linked by something that Buckminster Fuller called "Synergetics" and that there are symbolic analogies and affinities among various things of the same or similar vibration. This is reflected in the Hermetic maxim, "As above, so below; as below, so above." This principle affirms that a person affects one thing by changing something else that corresponds to it, including matter, energy, mind, and spirit. Thus, one can study and influence the unknown through the known or affect an action or thing through that which symbolizes it. The table of tarot correspondences on pages 42–43 indicates some of the general correspondences of the tarot to other symbols and systems. The correspondences to the essential oils are not included here, because they will be discussed in detail in the next few chapters.

Therefore, at one level, the tarot is a symbol-pigeonholing or memory system that interconnects related principles and experiences. In other words, the tarot can be used as a kind of information cataloguing device, a technique that I can personally attest to, having used the tarot very effectively this way for over fifty-five years. It is a development of the *Ars Memoria*, or "Art of Memory," that was elaborated by the 15th-century Platonist Renaissance philosopher Marcilio Ficino.

Because aromas are directly communicated to the brain, bypassing the cerebral cortex, they are also a direct link to your own emotions, memories, thoughts, and knowledge. Using both aroma and tarot together magically, as we shall see, gives us an incredibly powerful tool for personal growth, self-understanding, and for aligning ourselves with elemental forces that manifest in both the physical and metaphysical planes.

Symbols are often encoded in myths. As Sheryl Karas expresses it, "Ancient tales were created to teach the rules of the universe, as they were then understood, and the best ways to live according to those rules."[3] She sees the story of Adam and Eve as portraying the point at which humans became aware of themselves as separate from their environment, developing magic as a way to control what they no longer understood.

Oils and Scents as Symbols

There are many symbols on the tarot cards relating to essential oils (rose, lily, iris, acacia, cypress, etc.), as well as to other plants. Before we make our own associations between the cards and the oils, let's look at the significance of the traditional plant symbolism on the cards of the RWS deck.

Ivy appears on the robe of the **Fool**, indicating his relationship to Bacchus or Dionysus. Ivy represents life and abundance. The Fool's motley garb, with its sparks of fire and whirling wheels, represents the life force.

The white rose, representing purity and innocence, appears many times: first, in the hand of the **Fool**, where its fragrance is his guide; and **Death** carries a white rose on his banner. In both cards, it represents desire and passion—as do all roses—but, being white, is pure and innocent—the desire of the soul for perfection, passionately yearning for union with the Divine. On the Death card, in its perfect mandala shape, the rose also represents completion. Roses in general are a Hermetic sign of secrecy and silence. Supposedly a rose was given to Harpocrates, the god of silence (pictured on the Harris-Crowley Aeon card with finger to mouth), to keep him from revealing the secret of eternal life. It was, of course, the Great Goddess who gave him the rose, which represents her gift of sexuality as the source of all creation (and thus the secret of eternal life).

About the Tarot

TABLE OF TAROT CORRESPONDENCES

Card No.	Card Name	Hebrew Letter	Letter Meaning	Astro-logical	Music Note	Color	Gem	Animal	Magical Weapon
0	**Fool**	*Aleph*	Ox	Uranus	E	Pale Yellow	Tourmaline, Turquoise	Eagle, Man Butterfly	Dagger & Fan
1	**Magician**	*Beth*	House	Mercury	E	Yellow	Tiger Eye, Citrine, Fire Opal, Agate	Ibis, Ape, Swallow	Wand, Caduceus
2	**Priestess**	*Gimel*	Camel	Moon	G#	Blue	Moonstone, Pearl	Dog	Bow & Arrow
3	**Empress**	*Daleth*	Door	Venus	F#	Emerald Green	Emerald, Rose Quartz	Sparrow, Dove, Swan	Girdle or Belt
4	**Emperor**	*Heh*	Window	Aries	C	Scarlet Red	Ruby	Ram, Owl	Horns, Burin
5	**Hierophant**	*Vau*	Nail, Hook	Taurus	C#	Red-Orange	Topaz, Smoky Quartz, Carnelian, Lapis Lazuli	Bull	Labor of Preparation
6	**Lovers**	*Zain*	Sword	Gemini	D	Orange	Alexandrite, Agate	Magpie	Tripod
7	**Chariot**	*Cheth*	Fence	Cancer	D	Orange-Yellow	Amber, Chalcedony Carnelian	Sphinx, Crab, Turtle	Fiery Furnace
8	**Strength**	*Teth*	Serpent	Leo	E	Yellow	Cat's Eye, Topaz, Chrysolite	Lion	Discipline
9	**Hermit**	*Yod*	Hand (open)	Virgo	F	Yellow-Green	Peridot/Olivine, Bloodstone	Rhinoceros, Dog	Wand & Lamp
10	**Wheel of Fortune**	*Kaph*	Hand (closed)	Jupiter	A#	Royal Violet	Sapphire, Lapis, Amethyst	Eagle, Sphinx	Scepter

TABLE OF TAROT CORRESPONDENCES (continued)

Card No.	Card Name	Hebrew Letter	Letter Meaning	Astro-logical	Music Note	Color	Gem	Animal	Magical Weapon
11	**Justice**	*Lamed*	Ox Goad	Libra	F#	Emerald Green	Emerald, Coral, Jade	Elephant, Crane	Cross of Equilibrium
12	**Hanged One**	Mem	Water	Neptune	G#	Deep Blue	Aquamarine, Beryl	Snake, Eagle, Scorpion	Cup & Cross
13	**Death**	*Nun*	Fish	Scorpio	G	Blue-Green	Snakestone, Bloodstone	Wolf, Beetle, Crayfish	Evil Eye, Pain of Obligation
14	**Temperance**	*Samekh*	Prop	Sagit-tarius	G#	Blue	Jacinth, Amethyst	Horse, Dog, Centaur	Arrows
15	**Devil**	*Ayin*	Eye	Capricorn	A	Indigo	Black Diamond, Jet, Obsidian	Goat, Ass	Evil Eye, Lamp
16	**Tower**	*Peh*	Mouth	Mars	C	Scarlet Red	Ruby, Garnet, Hematite	Bear, Wolf, Horse	Two-edged Sword
17	**Star**	*Tzaddi*	Fish-Hook	Aquarius	A#	Violet	Turquoise, Rock Crystal	Peacock, Man, Eagle	Censer
18	**Moon**	*Qoph*	Back of Head	Pisces	B	Violet-Red	Milk Opal, Moonstone, Pearl	Dolphin, Fish, Scarab	Magic Mirror
19	**Sun**	*Resh*	Head	Sun	D	Orange	Diamond, Topaz, Heliotrope	Sparrowhawk, Lion	Bow & Arrow, Spear
20	**Judgement**	*Shin*	Tooth	Pluto	C	Red	Fire Opal, Malachite, Fire Agate	Lion	Wand, Lamp
21	**World**	*Tau*	Mark	Saturn	A	Blue-Violet	Onyx, Jet, Lapis Lazuli, Black Pearl	Crocodile, Dragon	Sickle

Red roses speak of instinct, passion, and the fiery spirit, while white lilies stand for intellect, purity, and the peaceful soul. In the legends of Mary's immaculate conception by her mother Anne, and again in her own immaculate conception of the Christ-child, it was the smelling of a rose and a lily, respectively, that achieved the miracles. These flowers usually appear together to balance the dual energies characterized as whore and maiden, sexuality and innocence, desire and intellect, imagination and will. Roses and lilies are the most prevalent plants in the RWS deck, adapted by Western magicians to represent the requirements of magic. The **Magician** must cultivate the five roses before him—representing the five senses (source of all desires)—as well as the four lilies representing the four elements (or worlds of abstract thought). The **Hierophant** recognizes these drives in his two acolytes, for the robe of one is covered in roses and the other in lilies, and as teacher, the Hierophant must speak to the needs of each.

Florence Farr, a chief in the Hermetic Order of the Golden Dawn from which the RWS deck evolved, explained in a work on plant alchemy the magical views represented by the rose and lily: "The sun and the moon are the Celestial luminaries, but the central ones are a fire hidden in the earth or nitre, and an airy lunar nature in the water. These two mixed natures are known to us as the desires of the flesh [rose] and the phantasies of the imagination [lily]: in their transmutation by consecration of the desires [rose] and purification of the thoughts [lily], lies the pathway to wisdom. The will [rose] and the imagination [lily] of an adept are symbolized by the Urim and Thummin of the High Priest."[4] The Urim and Thummin were oracular devices mentioned in the Old Testament for determining the will of God, worn by the high priest on his "breastplate of judgment"; in the Hierophant card they are symbolized by the rose and the lily.

These flowers also appear on several Minor Arcana cards: in the **2 of Wands**, the rose and lily are crossed, representing the choice facing the initiate. We return to the garden of the Magician in the **Ace of Pentacles**, where, with the knowledge gained on our journey through the tarot, we may choose to remain in the garden of earthly experience or leave through the gate into the unknown. Lilies supposedly sprang from the tears of Eve when she was expelled from the Garden, as memories of her lost innocence.

Additionally, red roses appear in **Strength** as a garland linking the maiden with the lion (her desire-nature); in a sense the maiden is the lily and the lion is the rose. Red roses formed like a Venus symbol (representing love) appear on the gown of the **Empress**, while red roses on the quilt of the **9 of Swords** promise that in time (symbolized by the checkerboard signs of the zodiac), the nightmare of depression will transform back into a desire for life.

Palm trees are embroidered on the veil behind the **High Priestess**. They are phallic symbols indicating archetypal masculine virility and also represent the spine. The pomegranates on the same veil symbolize female fertility (many seeds), the womb, and the heart. Their Hebrew name rimmon means "to bear a child." At least one tradition names pomegranates as the forbidden fruit in the Garden of Eden. (The Assyrian equivalent to palms and pomegranates was to alternate pinecones and lotuses.) Furthermore, from the gown of the High Priestess flows her liquid essence: as a symbol for the soul, she is the source of all essential oils.

Cypresses are symbolic of both death and rebirth. In **The Empress** card, they represent solace and comfort offered by a woman of maturity, and remind us how close birth is to death—that the new life the Empress carries is born to die.

The apple tree behind the woman on **The Lovers** card represents earthly desires and fecundity. Apples appear in many myths as a reward given to the woman of greatest allure and beauty, but it is always a reward with a price.

The flame-tree behind the man in the Lovers is the Tree of Life but aromatically could represent a resinous tree like the sacred frankincense or myrrh, burning its fragrant incense in sacrifice to the gods.

An ash tree, reminiscent of the World Tree, Yggdrasil, on which Odin hung himself, is featured on **The Hanged Man** card, where it represents magical sacrifice.

About the Tarot

The iris flower on the **Temperance** card represents Iris, the cup bearer of the gods and handmaiden of Hera, who, as the rainbow, was guide for the souls of women.

Traditionally the bush in the background of **The Star** card is an acacia, which has a long magical tradition. Sacred to the Egyptians, it represents reincarnation, the soul, and immortality. Since it blossoms simultaneously both white and red, it combines the symbolism of the red/white rose and the red rose/white lily. According to occultist Paul Foster Case, the bush represents the human brain and nervous system, and on it perches the ibis—the symbol of Thoth, the Egyptian god of learning and magic. Surrounding the pond are ten tiny flowers, which I believe are violets, since they represent the transitory qualities of life that are made apparent to us during mystical meditation; they also induce sleep. They may also represent the maidens transformed into flowers by Cupid to hide them from Aphrodite's jealousy of their beauty.

Sunflowers appear on **The Sun** card. They are abundant with seeds (which when pressed make an excellent carrier oil), representing the radiant energy of life that heliotropically turns towards the One. They also appear on the **Queen of Wands**, where the bold flower head represents haughtiness and pride, together with reasoned perception—the ability to shed light on all issues.

Evergreen wreaths appear frequently in the deck, and may be of myrtle or bay laurel. The Empress, Fool, and woman in the **2 of Cups** are probably crowned with myrtle wreaths, while the **Charioteer** and the champion in the **6 of Wands** are, more likely, wearing laurel wreaths. Additional wreaths depend from the wand of the victor in the **6 of Wands**, and arise from a cup in the **7 of Cups**. Myrtle was sacred to Aphrodite and Astarte, being a sign of immortality and promise of resurrection. To the Greeks, it was a sign of authority and used to crown bloodless victors. Awarded to poets, it signified that their fame would remain ever green. The laurel, on the other hand, was sacred to Apollo but similarly denoted victory, success, and fame everlasting. Additionally, it was associated with prophecy.

The wreath surrounding the dancer on **The World** card is, I believe, of myrtle. In older decks, this is a wreath of flowers representing the fragrant aura, the "odor of sanctity" mentioned earlier. Myrtle, sacred to the Goddess, was the chief scented tree in the Garden of Eden. According to an Arabic myth, God allowed Adam and Eve to take it with them so that its fragrance would remind them of resurrection, love, and immortality.

The garland of fruit and flowers in the **4 of Wands**—and the profusion of grapes, pumpkins, oranges, and apples in the **3 of Cups**—represents harvest, bounty, sharing, and fertility—as do the pears and apples in the **Queen of Pentacles**.

A palm frond and a sprig of myrtle (complete with berries) drape from the pierced crown of the **Ace of Swords**. The image here is of the Cabalistic Tree of Life—comprising ten sephiroth (or "spheres" of light)—of which the three highest are pictorially represented: Kether ("crown-indicated," literally), Chokmah (wisdom, and the Pillar of Mercy—indicated by the palm frond), and Binah (understanding, and the Pillar of Severity—indicated by the myrtle sprig). The sword itself signifies the middle pillar of the Tree. Historically, the palm was awarded to victorious gladiators in Rome and the myrtle to successful generals.

Water lilies appear in the **Ace of Cups** and on the robe of the **Page of Cups**. The Harris-Crowley Thoth deck features the water lily (lotus) on many of the cards. The water lily traditionally blends solar and lunar consciousness—the center is the sun (or son) surrounded by the feminine petals. Rooted in mud, it rises through the life-waters of the unconscious, and opens in the air to receive the life of the sun, which releases the flower's heavenly aroma. As the favorite scent of the Egyptians, the lotus represents the quintessence. Signifying creativity and spiritual evolution, in the Thoth deck especially, the state and color of the lotuses indicate the creative, vital, and spiritual state described by the particular card.

A mythical pentacle or "money bush" appears in the **7 of Pentacles**, but it looks nothing like the so-called money plant (lunaria). The reference

About the Tarot

here is to the patience and trust needed while waiting for the fruits of one's labors to ripen.

The **6 of Cups** features a kind of fantastical white star-flower in each cup (a giant star jasmine, a wild white rose, a white periwinkle?). But the images also represent the enclosed garden—as in the Song of Solomon (4:12), where: "A garden enclosed is my sister, my spouse, a spring shut up, a fountain sealed." The children are, at least metaphorically, brother and sister, and still innocent as the white flower implies. Interestingly, the enclosed garden of the **9 of Pentacles** represents with its hanging grapes the mature, voluptuous, and fertile female, while that of the **Ace of Pentacles** offers an open gateway to new experience.

Oak leaves, sacred to thunder-and-lightning gods like Zeus and Thor, top the helmet of the **Knight of Pentacles** (and his horse), indicating that he is the Oak King or Green Man. In Rome, oak leaves were a sign of service to the state or awarded for saving the life of a citizen, portraying endurance and strength.

Bunches of grapes and vines of grape leaves are found on the robes of the **King of Pentacles** and the old man in the **10 of Pentacles**. The wall of the **9 of Pentacles** is also covered in grapes. Grapes are ambivalent. They represent both fertility/new life, and blood/sacrifice. In these three cards, they depict wealth and a rich, full life—but with a hint of recognition that this is merely a fleeting experience in the face of deeper truths. The additional meaning of intoxication does not always apply here.

Finally, two small red flowers blossom on the tree of life in the stained glass window in the **5 of Pentacles**, promising that spring will follow the cold of winter.

Two Major Arcana cards refer especially to essential oils—**Temperance** and **The Star**.

The Temperance card represents an angel who is also an alchemist (the Thoth deck makes this clear by calling its card Art), mixing the Elixir of Life from the essential oils of plants. This involves not only distillation but synergy; that is, combining oils to make entirely new molecular structures, each with their own subtle effect. The mystery of how water can flow sideways is solved when we realize that it is actually the essential aromas that are being "poured" like smoke from vessel to vessel.

The Star card shows clearly the ethereal and meditative state that can be produced by a suitably fragrant atmosphere. In fact, most scents are strongest at night. They are also, like the figure in the card, "truth" unveiled from its material form. We see here how scent can provide a link between the universal macrocosm and the planetary microcosm, and how it can help us perceive the underlying patterns of the cosmos. The peacock sometimes appears on The Star card (see especially the *Aquarian Tarot* by David Palladini), and is suggestive of essential oils and perfumes because of its iridescent, opulent beauty—which also symbolizes the glory of the immortal soul. The tail feathers of the peacock were made into fans used in certain Moorish countries and some south European courts to waft fragrances through the air, and its beak was used in Persia and later in Europe to spray scent. The "magical weapon" or tool assigned to The Star card by the Golden Dawn was the incense censor.

CHAPTER 4

Imagination and Aroma Imaging

*"Scents are surer than sounds or sights to
make your heart strings crack."*
—Rudyard Kipling, 1865–1936

The Nature of Olfaction

It is intriguing that, although aromatic correspondences (to planets and signs of the zodiac, gems, metals, spirits, and tarot cards, etc.) have remained remarkably consistent through the ages, an individual's emotional reactions and aromatic associations have no predictability. Some reactions are cultural, and some are entirely personal. For instance, in some cultures the smell of garlic or cabbage enhances the sense of pleasure in eating, while in others it is repellant. While some people associate the smell of vanilla with a mother's warmth and nurturance; others find it cloying and trivial. Costly and treasured spikenard, used to anoint the feet of Jesus, smells fetid to some people today—unpleasantly like "muck." Many people find that pine reminds them of grammar school bathrooms rather than a mountain forest.

Cynthia Giles, in her book *The Tarot: History, Mystery, and Lore*, speculates that "potent images, such as those of the Tarot, could serve as tuning devices for the brain." This can also be said, of course, about scents—and this is one way that we will be using both tarot and essential oils. Giles continues with a discussion of the largely ignored existence of covert awareness. "This term," she says, "describes perception, memory, and judgment carried out *unconsciously*—in other words, the structure and process of what you know, but don't know that you know"[1]—that is, how your senses provide information of which you are consciously unaware.

Bear with me now as I take you through a different and ultimately magical look at olfactory activity and covert awareness in the brain. Science is now acknowledging a macro view of perception (along with the micro view of neuron activity) that has led to the discovery in the brain of *chaos*. Chaos is here defined as "complex behavior that seems random [i.e., changeable] but actually has some hidden order," as explained by Walter J. Freeman in his report to *Scientific American* describing studies of the olfactory system.[2] He gives, as an example of chaos, commuters dashing about in a train station—where *order* underlies the surface complexity versus the *randomness* of a terrified crowd. When a change of track is announced in a "chaotic" train station, there is a definite change of movement. This sounds remarkably like Carl Jung's concept of synchronicity, in which things happening at the same time are meaningfully related although we cannot see the connection on the surface. Primarily, chaos allows the brain to respond flexibly and generate new patterns of activity.

When someone smells a particular odor, it is not only recognized in the olfactory bulb (before it gets to the limbic brain or any other part of the brain), but *"the bulb participates in assigning meaning."*[3] This has been demonstrated in the laboratory, where amplitude maps representing a given odorant change strikingly when the reinforcement associated with the scent (that is, "meaning based on experience") is altered. What this demonstrates is that the earliest recognitions of different scents in the brain are not to the scent itself but to *what one associates with it!*

Additionally, training strengthens sensitivity at the synaptic level among all the neurons (even those connected with other parts of the brain) that were simultaneously excited during learning. In other words, synapses that fire together are strengthened together—if rewarded for doing so. This process is affected by two things: 1) arousal through fear and desire (modified by brain chemicals, among them hormones), and 2) continued input after initial excitation of the neurons. "If the odorant is familiar and the bulb has been primed by arousal," says Freeman, "the information spreads like a flash fire. First, excitatory input to one part during a sniff excites the other parts. . . . Then those parts re-excite the first . . . so that the input rapidly ignites an explosion of collective activity . . . [which], in turn, spreads to the entire bulb, igniting a full-blown burst."[4] The outer evidence of this inner burst can be the sudden experience of being in another time and place with all attendant emotions fully present.

Self-organization is a characteristic of chaotic systems and depends on flexibility and the ability to generate new patterns in order to make dramatic changes, even when the input is weak. The limbic system (which is involved in emotion and memory and is itself a self-organized chaotic system) gives a command to the senses to gather information. "Synchronous activity in each system is then transmitted back to the limbic system, where it combines with similarly generated output from other sensory systems to form a gestalt, only to begin again."[5] Thus brains grow, reorganize themselves, and reach into their environment to change it to their own advantage. "As above, so below." This, Freeman believes, may be what we call consciousness. In an associative memory system, new learning will, to a greater or lesser degree, affect *all* previous learning. So too with smells. Learning a new smell (actually a memory and emotion keyed to a smell) affects your reaction to all previous smells. If you associate the scent of eucalyptus with being cared for by your mother when you were ill, then later experiences in a eucalyptus forest will modify that initial pattern but also will subtly affect all your other experiences with smells. Magic, which has been defined as the ability to change consciousness at will, essentially has the same kind of repatterning ability.

Imagination and Aroma Imaging

Aroma and Imagination

Still, it takes more than just the mechanisms of the brain to create magic. As we will see, it takes will, desire, and imagination. Edwin T. Morris in his book *Fragrance* discovered that perfumers speak eloquently about imagination. He quotes Edmond Roudnitska, maker of perfumes for the house of Dior, as saying, "The capacity to create is *essentially* the ability to imagine." Morris adds, "It is imagination that enables the creator to take reality and twist it into the work of art. As Gaston Bachelard notes, imagination is that which is able to 'give a new form to the world' by '*deforming* images provided by perception.' He likens it to a great tree, at home in both the earth and the sky."[6]

Smell is the premier sense for making us think. It works on the mind; it changes your mood; it breaks down limitations.

Magician Florence Farr said that magic was the ability to "unlimit experience"—which is essential if we are to "deform perceptions" in order to reform the world. As Cynthia Giles explains in her exploration of the tarot, ordinary perception is bound by the material world through the senses. Imagination, however, is free of the rules of time and space that govern materiality. Because the imagination is so vast and powerful, it is both seductive and frightening. Thus, people have been frightened by the seductive power of scent through the ages—afraid that it might disturbingly "unlimit" their known world. It is the poets, shamans, mystics, artists, magicians, and, may I add, perfumers, who do, as Giles calls it, "imaginary reconnaissance." They venture into the wild places of the imagination and create maps and signposts to guide others. "Imagination," she says, "is the faculty that allows us to experience the immaterial."[7]

Aroma Imaging with Tarot Oils

We have seen that smells are recognized (and electrically imprinted in the brain) by the associations, conscious and unconscious, that you make to them. These imprints carry the emotional weight of your feelings at the time, and they also trigger your hormones, immune system, breathing pattern and heartbeat, body temperature, insulin production, appetite, thirst, digestion, sexual arousal, and nerves! At its most simplistic level, offensive odors make you impatient and irritable. Pleasant odors revive you so that you feel bright and cheery. Strong concentrates of certain scents are disagreeable, sometimes highly oppressive, and can even cause you to faint. While there is a certain predictability about how and which scents will affect you, your individual reactions or deliberate training can override these generalized predilections.

The important thing is that you can consciously control your responses to scents! I call this "aroma imaging," which is a way of consciously patterning your aromatic responses via the systematic use of tarot oils and tarot cards. We know that scents serendipitously produce any kind of memory recall, depending on your individual experiences; for example, a bright spring day could be evoked by the scent of gasoline, or fear of punishment by the scent of chalk, or a math equation by the smell of lilacs that once bloomed at the classroom window. It's easy to see how much more useful to us those scents could be if we deliberately created memories and emotional states by using what we know about symbolic correspondences.

As aromatherapist Valerie Ann Worwood points out in her book *Aromantics*, we sometimes need "reprogramming."[8] If you associate lavender with a grandmother who was always ill and crotchety, then you can change that association by creating a beautiful environment of your favorite music, a warm bath, the company of a friend, and indulge yourself with some pleasurable, youthful activity while wearing lavender oil or spraying it through the air with a diffuser. It may take several sessions, but eventually you will find yourself looking forward to your "lavender times." Or, if you enjoy the outdoors, find someone with a patch of lavender (or plant your own), and, on a beautiful warm day go sit in the midst of it, crush the flowers between your fingers and meditate on the beauty and unity of life. Think only pleasant thoughts, associate yourself with the earth energies, and even speak to the plant and listen to what it has to teach you.

Imagination and Aroma Imaging

While you are sitting with the plants, or in a pleasantly scented room, notice how your depth of breathing increases, how your lungs slowly but powerfully fill and empty, as you attempt to draw in as much of the aroma to your olfactory center as you can. When in the presence of pleasant fragrances, we breathe more deeply, become more aware of the environment, and increase blood and oxygen circulation to the brain and throughout the body. This is one way in which essential oils can improve health, stimulate awareness and imagination, and create calmness and serenity. Conversely, in the presence of unpleasant odors (or unpleasant associations to them), you become anxious and naturally tend to hold back your breathing, which becomes shorter and shallower. It protects your life force but restricts your consciousness.

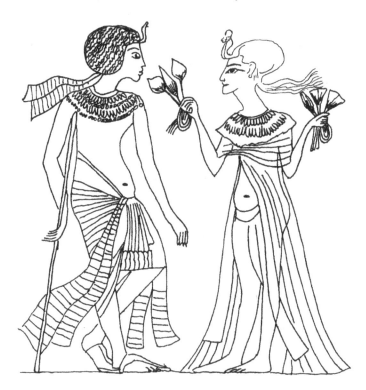

When you reprogram your associations—or as I prefer to call it, when you do aroma imaging—you should try to expand your awareness to include the whole range of possible associations to the oils. Take into account all the physiological effects that the oils produce. Recall their archetypal meanings and their symbolic associations with myths and legends, goddesses and gods. Think about their uses as revealed by tradition, folklore, and folk magic—these often create a link between medicinal effects and the collective unconscious.

Next are the associations based on what is called the "doctrine of signatures"—which is often at the root of traditional lore. Paracelsus taught that "all things have their stamp or signature and that signature is a clue to their connectedness to other things with similar signatures."[9] Resins oozing from a tree were thought to help with open wounds; vines were thought to relate to veins; red plants and flowers were related to the red planet Mars and to blood, and thence to rage and passion. Such associations are, as the author and occultist E. E. Rehmus explains, based on the principle of the essential unity of man and cosmos.[10] They are not mumbo-jumbo, but pragmatic linkages upon which to forge alliances of memory and magical power and are the basis for traditional correspondences.

The Tarot Oils

The tarot oils are essential-oil synergies usually consisting of two to four individual oils that correspond primarily to the twenty-two Major Arcana of the tarot and, less specifically, to the number and people cards of the Minor Arcana. When combined with a "carrier oil" such as almond, olive, or jojoba oil, they can be used for self-anointing and for working with the tarot cards and their energies. Ideally, you will eventually create your own entire set of twenty-two tarot oils, but, practically speaking, you will want to begin with the oils for only two or three cards. One way of doing this is to work first with the essential oils corresponding to your own personality and soul cards. Appendix A tells you how to determine your special tarot cards based on your birthdate.

Imagination and Aroma Imaging

Tarot oils are powerful tools for aroma imaging because they link the symbology of the oils with the corresponding symbology of the tarot cards, creating evocative emotional-memory links between the two. It's a smell/sight imagination punch of tremendous power! The symbols of the Major Arcana are keyed to traditional correspondences, and to innumerable myths and stories, old and new. You can mimic them through movement and dance and use affirmations associated with them as chants and songs of power. Although incense and anointing oils have been used for thousands of years, odor is still the missing link in most modern attempts to repattern, empower, or initiate people. Scents build confidence and self-esteem. They should be one of your greatest tools for achieving whatever goals you set.

Many of the rituals and techniques given later in this book are about consciously imaging what you want using the scents of the tarot oils and the pictures on the tarot cards.

CHAPTER 5

The Tarot Oils

*"When we accept small wonders,
we qualify ourselves to imagine great wonders."*
—Tom Robbins, *Jitterbug Perfume*

Astrological Correspondences

There is a long tradition for associating plants and essential oils with goddesses, gods, and astrological signs that exists in some form in almost every country on the planet. Before giving you my choices for oils that can be combined to form the tarot oils, I suggest you review the following chart, which associates the essential oils with elements and astrological signs and planets. These correspondences are generally based on attributions traditional to Western European magic and are similar although not identical to the attributions by the Hermetic Order of the Golden Dawn, the Wiccan fairy tradition, 17th-century astrologer/herbalist Nicholas Culpeper, and contemporary magical aromatherapist Scott Cunningham. They represent several years of experimentation on my part and are open to further revision.

For the botanical names of the plants used in the oils, refer to the individual tarot oil descriptions or to their names in Appendix B: Master Chart of the Essential Oils.

ASTROLOGICAL CORRESPONDENCES: ELEMENTS, PLANETS, AND SIGNS

An asterisk * indicates that the oil appears in more than one category within that section.

ELEMENTS

Fire Angelica, Basil, Bay Laurel, Bergamot*, Black Pepper, Carrot*, Cedar, Cinnamon, Clove, Coriander*, Cumin*, Frankincense, Ginger*, Hyssop, Juniper Berry, Mandarin, Neroli, Nutmeg, Orange, Pennyroyal*, Pettigrain, Rosemary, Rue, Saffron, Sassafras.

Water Camphor, Cardamom*, Carrot*, Chamomile, Coriander*, Cumin*, Cypress*, Geranium*, Ginger*, Honeysuckle, Jasmine, Labdanum, Lemon, Marjoram*, Melissa, Mugwort, Myrrh, Opoponax, Pennyroyal*, Sandalwood, Spikenard*, Valerian, Vanilla*, Ylang-ylang.

Air Anise, Bergamot*, Caraway*, Chamomile (Blue), Clary Sage*, Dill, Eucalyptus, Fennel, Fir, Geranium*, Lavender, Lemongrass, Lime, Marjoram*, Myrtle*, Niaouli, Palmarosa, Peppermint, Pine, Rose*, Sage*, Spearmint, Storax, Thyme*.

Earth Balsam de Peru, Bois de Rose, Caraway*, Cardomom*, Clary Sage*, Cypress*, Myrtle*, Narcissus, Oakmoss, Patchouli, Rose*, Sage*, Spikenard*, Thyme*, Vanilla*, Vetivert, Wintergreen.

PLANETS

Sun Angelica, Bay Laurel*, Bergamot*, Carrot*, Cedar*, Cinnamon, Frankincense, Juniper Berry, Lime*, Mandarin, Neroli, Orange, Rosemary.

Moon Camphor, Chamomile (Roman and Blue*), Honeysuckle*, Jasmine, Labdanum, Lemon, Mugwort, Myrrh*, (also many white, night-blooming, tropical flowers).

Mercury Anise*, Caraway, Clary Sage*, Dill, Eucalyptus*, Fennel, Lavender*, Lemongrass, Narcissus, Peppermint, Sage*, Spearmint, Storax, Thyme*, Wintergreen.

Venus Balsam de Peru, Bois de Rose, Cardamom, Cypress*, Geranium, Lavender*, Marjoram, Myrtle, Oakmoss*, Palmarosa, Patchouli*, Rose, Sandalwood*, Thyme*, Vanilla, Vetivert, Ylang-ylang.

Mars Basil, Black Pepper, Carrot*, Coriander*, Cumin, Ginger, Pennyroyal*, Pettigrain, Pine, Rue, Sassafras.

Jupiter Bay Laurel*, Bergamot*, Cedar*, Clove*, Hyssop, Melissa*, Nutmeg, Saffron, Sage*, Sandalwood*.

Saturn Clary Sage*, Cypress*, Eucalyptus*, Fir, Myrrh*, Oakmoss*, Patchouli*, Spikenard*, Vetivert.

Uranus Chamomile (Blue)*, Eucalyptus*, Fennel*, Lime*, Niaouli.

Neptune Honeysuckle*, Melissa*, Mugwort*. Myrrh*, Sandalwood*, Spikenard*.

Pluto Anise*, Basil*, Cypress*, Opoponax, Pennyroyal*, Valerian.

ASTROLOGICAL CORRESPONDENCES: ELEMENTS, PLANETS, AND SIGNS (continued)

An asterisk * indicates that the oil appears in more than one category within that section.

SIGNS OF THE ZODIAC

Aries
(Cardinal Fire, ruled by Mars, Sun exalted)
Bay Laurel, Black Pepper, Cedar*, Frankincense*, Ginger*, Pettigrain, Pine*, Rue, Sassafras.

Taurus
(Fixed Earth, ruled by Venus, Moon exalted)
Bois de Rose, Cardamom, Geranium, Jasmine*, Myrtle*, Oakmoss*, Patchouli*, Rose, Thyme*, Vanilla*.

Gemini
(Mutable Air, ruled by Mercury)
Dill, Eucalyptus*, Fennel*, Lavender*, Lemongrass, Peppermint, Spearmint*, Storax.

Cancer
(Cardinal Water, ruled by Moon, Jupiter exalted)
Camphor, Carrot, Chamomile, Honeysuckle*, Jasmine*, Labdanum*, Lemon.

Leo
(Fixed Fire, ruled by Sun)
Bay Laurel, Cinnamon, Frankincense*, Juniper Berry, Mandarin, Neroli, Rosemary, Saffron*.

Virgo
(Mutable Earth, ruled by Mercury, Mercury exalted)
Caraway, Clary Sage*, Narcissus, Spikenard*, Wintergreen.

Libra
(Cardinal Air, ruled by Venus, Saturn exalted)
Cypress, Lavender*, Marjoram*, Myrtle*, Niaouli*, Palmarosa*, Rose, Spearmint*, Thyme*.

Scorpio
(Fixed Water, ruled by Mars and Pluto, Uranus exalted)
Anise*, Basil, Coriander, Cumin, Cypress*, Ginger*, Labdanum*, Opoponax, Pennyroyal, Pine*, Rue, Valerian.

Sagittarius
(Mutable Fire, ruled by Jupiter)
Angelica, Bergamot, Cedar*, Clove, Coriander*, Hyssop, Nutmeg, Sage, Saffron*.

Capricorn
(Cardinal Earth, ruled by Saturn, Mars exalted)
Clary Sage*, Oakmoss*, Patchouli*, Spikenard*, Vetivert.

Aquarius
(Fixed Air, ruled by Saturn and Uranus)
Chamomile (Blue), Clary Sage*, Eucalyptus*, Fennel*, Fir, Lime, Niaouli*.

Pisces
(Mutable Water, ruled by Jupiter and Neptune, Venus exalted)
Honeysuckle*, Marjoram*, Melissa, Mugwort, Myrrh*, Sandalwood*, Spikenard*, Ylang-ylang.

Choosing the Oils to Work With

You may select oils for your own magical use by using the lists of astrological correspondences to the oils in the preceding chart. But be aware that several principles are involved, as suggested by the information in the following chart: Oils corresponding to your sun and moon sign, or their rulers (as in, Venus rules *Libra*, etc.) are good for "signature" scents that represent your most strongly radiant qualities, and they are an excellent basis for combinations that will draw others to you. However, if you are selecting oils to bring out latent qual-

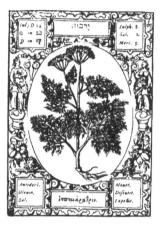

ities in yourself or to redress or balance your own natural proclivities, these won't do at all. Then you will want to draw from the signs and their rulers that are opposite your own. Use the list below to help you "balance" your energies with oils selected according to their astrological rulerships and oppositions.

ASTROLOGICAL RULERSHIPS AND OPPOSITIONS

— opposed to —

Aries is ruled by **Mars**	*Libra* is ruled by **Venus**
Taurus is ruled by **Venus**	*Scorpio* is ruled by **Mars** and **Pluto**
Gemini is ruled by **Mercury**	*Sagittarius* is ruled by **Jupiter**
Cancer is ruled by the **Moon**	*Capricorn* is ruled by **Saturn**
Leo is ruled by the **Sun**	*Aquarius* is ruled by **Saturn** and **Uranus**
Virgo is ruled by **Mercury**	*Pisces* is ruled by **Jupiter** and **Neptune**

The two zodiacal signs ruled by the same planet also have opposing characteristics.

— ruler —

(Earth)	*Capricorn*	**Saturn**	*Aquarius*	(Air)
(Fire)	*Sagittarius*	**Jupiter**	*Pisces*	(Water)
(Water)	*Scorpio*	**Mars**	*Aries*	(Fire)
(Air)	*Libra*	**Venus**	*Taurus*	(Earth)
(Earth)	*Virgo*	**Mercury**	*Gemini*	(Air)
(Fire)	*Leo*	**Sun/Moon**	*Cancer*	(Water)

Essence of Tarot

The Major Arcana Tarot Oils

Each new book on aromatherapy seems to contain dozens of new essential oils, not all of which can be found with ease even through the major distributors, much less in your local health-food store. The seventy oils described here to be used with tarot symbolism are generally available. Many of them should be relatively easy to find at a good health-food store or online at a reasonable price. Be aware that a few of the oils are quite expensive. Add them to your work when you want that "something extra." Expensive oils can be bought in amounts as small as one milliliter (20 to 25 drops), but they are so concentrated that you should then dilute them with about three to five times the amount of jojoba oil (it won't go rancid like other oils) before using them.

Each of the following tarot oils is a synergistic blend of the constituent oils described in the section that covers each card. Whether formed singly or in combination, they are all a continual work in progress! You may want to begin with a single essential oil for each card and then add others after a period of use. As you learn more about essential oils, feel free to modify or change the combinations I describe here. Although carefully worked out on the basis of my personal findings and inclinations, they are, after all, intended primarily to stimulate your own explorations—and are definitely not to be considered as graven in stone for the ages.

Tarot cards have complex, even paradoxical, natures. They do not, for instance, correspond exactly to the astrological signs and planets with which they are often associated (a different system—for example, one in which Saturn corresponds to The Hermit—may offer important insights). Usually, more than one essential oil is necessary to replicate the intricacy of a Major Arcana card. The first oil mentioned will always be a relatively inexpensive option and a good start for building your tarot oil set. In the chart below, any oil whose name is bracketed and in italics, thus: *[Jasmine]*, is an expensive oil that is not absolutely required but offers some special quality that may, on occasion, be worth the extra cost. Occasionally a cheaper alternative is suggested, or the flower essence may be used to access the finer subtle vibrations that such an oil can add.

The Tarot Oils

When experimenting with essential oils, research their physiological effects in addition to their emotional or traditional magical associations, for occasionally you will find these purposes in conflict; they might even cancel each other out. But remember that the magical use of oils differs from the medical and therapeutic uses. For magic and ritual, you will focus on applying the symbolism found in myth and folklore—which is generally ignored in therapeutic applications. In other words, you should assume that the old tales are metaphoric keys to the subtle effects of the oils pertaining to your spiritual essence; this is magical awareness as compared to a physical one.

	THE 22 MAJOR ARCANA TAROT OILS			
	Arcanum	**Constituents of the Major Arcana Tarot Oils**		
0	**Fool**	Fennel	Niaouli	—	—
1	**Magician**	Dill	Lemongrass	Storax	—
2	**High Priestess**	Camphor	Lemon	—	[Jasmine]
3	**Empress**	Ylang-ylang	Vanilla (Balsam)	★	[Rose]
4	**Emperor**	Ginger	Petitgrain	Bay Laurel	—
5	**Hierophant**	Thyme	Cardamom	Bois de Rose	—
6	**Lovers**	Lavender	Geranium	Peppermint	—
7	**Chariot**	Coriander	Carrot	Labdanum	[Chamomile (Roman)]
8	**Strength**	Rosemary	Juniper Berry	(Orange)	[Neroli]
9	**Hermit**	Sage	Wintergreen	Caraway	[Narcissus]
10	**Wheel of Fortune**	Cedar	Nutmeg	Clove	[Saffron]
11	**Justice**	Myrtle	Palmarosa	Spearmint	—
12	**Hanged One**	Mugwort	Spikenard	Myrrh	—
13	**Death**	Cypress	Rue (Valerian, Cumin)	—	[Opoponax]
14	**Temperance**	Hyssop	Bergamot	—	[Angelica]
15	**Devil**	Clary Sage	Patchouli	—	—
16	**Tower**	Black Pepper	Pine	Sassafras	—
17	**Star**	Eucalyptus	Fir	Lime	[Chamomile (Blue)]
18	**Moon**	Sandalwood	Marjoram	—	[Melissa]
19	**Sun**	Cinnamon	Mandarin	Frankincense	—
20	**Judgement**	Basil	Pennyroyal	Anise	—
21	**World**	Vetivert	Oakmoss	—	—
	*Rose Geranium or Palmarosa may be added to Empress Oil for the rose scent.				

Consider slowly building up your own set of individual oils through working with only those oils that most relate to your needs right now. As mentioned before, a good place to start is with the "key oils" that correspond to your personality and soul cards (see appendix A), or pick an oil corresponding to the planet that rules your sun, moon, or rising sign (see the preceding charts). Talk to your chosen oil and get to know it.

Important Warnings

Check the Latin names when purchasing oils to be sure you have what you want. Do not use synthetics. Never use these oils internally or on mucous membranes.[1] Always dilute your oils in a carrier oil or water (like a bath) or diffuse through the air, for many of them can be skin irritants when used at full strength. These potential skin irritants are marked with a single exclamation point in the text [!]. If you get a rash or feel a burning sensation, wash with cold water and then apply plain vegetable oil to disperse the effect. Oils that can be toxic in large doses; hazardous to epileptics, pregnant women, those who are allergic or sensitive; or which can cause headaches are marked with a double exclamation point [!!] following the Latin name. Do not use these oils undiluted directly on the skin.[2] The citruses make the skin more sensitive to harmful effects from the sun (photosensitive), so avoid them before and during outdoor experiences. If you are pregnant, use only the most gentle oils—such as lavender, chamomile, rose, jasmine, melissa, neroli, tangerine, and rose geranium. And lavender, chamomile, and tangerine are the only oils I'd recommend for children. Otherwise, diluted to the suggested dosages, all the oils below can be safely used for magical anointing. Some oils, such as peppermint and camphor, are antidotes to homeopathic remedies, so don't even store them near your remedies.

The Tarot Oils

Each card in the Major Arcana has specific astrological correspondences according to the Hermetic Order of the Golden Dawn, as do their oils. These correspondences follow the card's or oil's title and are ordered as follows:

- Primary element (plus /secondary element when a planet rules two zodiac signs)
- Ruling planet (plus secondary ruling planet, if applicable) of a zodiac sign
- Primary correspondence (final item): either a planet or a zodiac sign

Note that not every card has all three.

0—The Fool (Air, Uranus)

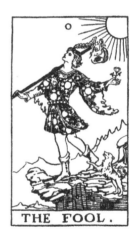

The Fool represents your spirit before manifestation and between incarnations. You are at a jumping-off point in life. You make the right choice when you don't mind looking foolish but act with joy, strength, and vitality—and, above all, with divine nonchalance. It is a time to take risks, for limitations are temporarily removed from your path. You need to get in touch with the child within yourself and to feel rejuvenated. As the Fool, others see you as a carefree vagabond relishing every moment of life, but you "foolishly" seem to forget or abandon each person or thing as the next one attracts your attention. They can't appreciate the Fool's ability to "be here now" without the usual baggage of guilt, limitations, and anxieties.

Fennel (*Foeniculum vulgare*)[!]—(Air, Mercury and Uranus as the higher vibration of Mercury)

This is a youthful energy promoting longevity—the Peter Pan effect. It promotes the courage to trust and to give unconditionally. Fennel expels "wind" (indigestive gas)—and the word folly comes from "windbag." It eliminates excess, for the Fool needs to be free, granting a sense of weightlessness. The poet Longfellow admired this tall herb that inhabits cliffs and hillsides: "Above the lower plants it towers/ The fennel with its yellow flowers/ And in an earlier age than ours/ Was gifted with the wondrous powers/ Lost vision to restore," and so the Fool sees everything as if for the first time. According to Sophocles, Prometheus brought the spark of fire down from Heaven hidden within a fennel stalk—just as the free spirit descends into manifestation hidden within the human body. It brings a sense of vitality and renewed trust in your opportunities for fully experiencing life.

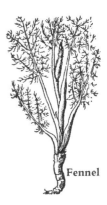
Fennel

Niaouli (*Melaleuca viridiflora*)—includes Cajeput, MQV (true niaouli—an acronym for its Latin name *Melaleuca quinquenervia viridiflora*), and Tea Tree—(Air, Uranus)

Niaouli frees us from the effects of physical forces and instincts. The Fool dances lightly at the edge of disaster yet is protected. Niaouli is like the little white dog that keeps the Fool from going over the edge. It is sharp and clean like the mountain air. It concentrates us in the present, diminishing the limiting awareness of past and future. Magician Scott Cunningham sees it as providing protection from psychic attack, but it is more like being so focused on the pure life force that nothing else can touch you.

The Tarot Oils

1—The Magician (Air/Earth, Mercury)

The Magician represents the state of focused consciousness. It is the awareness of yourself as a unique, creative individual, using your mind and will to channel your intent into actuality, manifesting idea into form. This is your ability to innovate, concentrate, and communicate your thoughts—transforming mundane situations into magical ones. When you embody the Magician energy, others see you as an independent leader, working solo, on your own initiative but perhaps unscrupulous about manipulating others to your way of thinking. Magicians can become cunning tricksters or con artists, creating

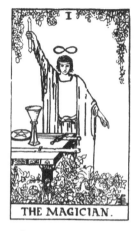

illusions to serve personal ends. On the other hand, as the Magician, you can be a networker and facilitator who acts as a catalyst for change. Under this influence, you are imaginative and skillful, and cultivate your environment as an expression of your uniqueness. The Magician represents the skill and ability—the power—to do things by yourself.

Dill (Anethum graveolens)—(Air, Mercury, Gemini)
Dill has a dominant personality. Roman gladiators rubbed it on their skins before arena combat because it sharpens the senses and heightens awareness of the environment. Warriors returning to Rome were crowned with garlands of dill; they then hung them in the banquet halls to stimulate their appetites. The word *dill* is Norse and means "to lull," thus "dilly" water or pillows have been used to sooth fidgety children and put colicky babies to sleep. In magical work, it protects children from roving malicious spirits. Dill

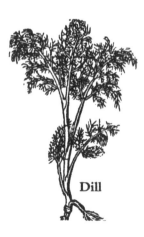

Essence of Tarot

focuses the mind for detail work and helps you to express yourself clearly and precisely. Lifting you to a more expanded form of consciousness, it brings objectivity to all your dealings. It expands the intellect and helps you to assimilate experiences and digest psychic and mental influences. Hildegard of Bingen praised its ability to suppress sexual impulses (important in a convent or when spending much time alone).

Lemongrass (*Cymbopogon citratus*)[!]—(Air, Mercury, Gemini)
With its sedating action on the nervous system, it soothes headaches, fights tiredness (good on long trips), and stimulates the thyroid. It is refreshing and radiant. Lemongrass stimulates left-brain and logical thinking and tightens connective tissue as well as connective thoughts. It helps you process new ideas. Use it to help in spirit communication, too.

Storax **(or *Styrax*)** (*Liquidambar orientalis or styraciflua*)—(Air, Mercury, Gemini)
Used to fumigate rooms and fix perfumes, Aleister Crowley said, "Storax is chiefly Mercurial on account of its nondescript nature, a menstruum for other perfumes in the same way as Mercury is the basis of amalgams." It is a mental stimulant and nervine, and is used in magic for creative work, money gain, and business activity.

Or, alternately: ***Benzoin*** (*Styrax benzoin, S. tonkinensis*)—(Air, Mercury, Gemini). Related to storax, benzoin was used as "holy smoke" among the Malays to ward off devils and was also burned at their rice harvesting ceremonies. In India, it was sacred to the Trimurti godhead, the trinity of Hindu deities. Also called "Friar's Balsam" or "gum benjamin," it is a tonic for the respiratory system and is also effective against itching of the skin. Psychically, it creates a protective shield, bringing forth dreams and poetry. It is energizing and warming, provoking sensual thoughts and releasing tensions and resentments. Use it for penetrating the depths of consciousness and bringing things safely to the consciousness, where you can objectively examine what has been irritating or annoying you.

The Tarot Oils

2—The High Priestess (Water, Moon)

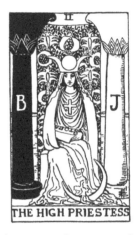

The High Priestess represents your deepest inner wisdom. She sits in the temple of your subconscious, nonjudgmentally contemplating (observing but not affected by) all your memories, feelings, inner tides of hormones and instincts, and sensory data. This vast awareness flows through her before emerging into your physical experience. But she only speaks through metaphors, appearing in dream symbols, memory images, emotions, and bodily reactions. You must look carefully at the symbolic meanings of these messages or, in quiet meditation, enter her temple and ask for advice.

When you embody her energy, others sense in you the power of mystery and inner-feminine wisdom. You feel yourself to be a vessel of oracular knowledge, influenced by lunar tides and cycles of inner knowing, more potent than mundane reason.

Camphor (*Cinnamomum camphora*) [!]—(Water, Moon, Cancer)
Aleister Crowley said, "The white waxen appearance suggests Luna, so also the perfume is peculiarly cleanly." Camphor is generally cooling, but its effects vary like the moon, according to the state of the person. It cools ardor and emotions, allowing you to dispassionately observe your involvements. When distilled, it forms solid crystalline memory cells. Its sharp odor sets up a pathway to your deep memories, your past lives, collective as well as personal, but it also veils them to protect you from their effects. Camphor cleanses your inner space of emotionality and rids you (temporarily) of psychic "pests." Too much of this effect brings headaches as the "pests" rush to evacuate your space.

Lemon (*Citrus limonum*)[!]—(Water, Moon, Cancer)
Lemon revitalizes, cleanses, purifies, and aids in healing by stimulating white corpuscles to fight off infection. While fresh and lively, it is also sedating and relaxing, helping you to maintain poise and calm. It will assist you in concentrating and thinking clearly during emotional turmoil and can aid in decision-making by breaking through mental blocks. It is cooling and virginal like the pale light of the moon, creating emotional space. Use it for maintaining independence and objectivity while working intuitively and psychically.

Jasmine[3] (*Jasminum grandiflorum*)—(Water, Moon, Cancer)

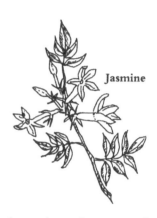

Jasmine

In India, jasmine is the flower of Lakshmi, the goddess of luck, happiness, and fortune and is called "Moonlight of the Grove." Also called "Mistress of the Night," it is a recognized aphrodisiac but refers magically to the spiritualization of sexuality. Jasmine awakens the spirit within the inner temple of the self, representing the sacred prostitute (*hetaera*) who belongs to no one but herself, the spirit who channels the love of the Divine so that the recipient may know the perfect union of opposites. Thus jasmine has the power to transcend earthly love. It grants a sense of wholeness and bolsters your self-confidence in relating to others. It also helps you access your own inner wisdom by awakening you to symbols and metaphors that can vitalize your imagination and intuition. The Mistress of the Night lifts your spirits, relieves depression, heightens spiritual awareness, brings psychic dreams, and treats emotionally based sexual dysfunctions. Jasmine is the essence of mystery and magic.

3—The Empress (Earth/Air, Venus)

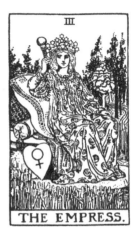

The Empress is the source of the creative life force and represents the fruitfulness of the earth. She is the earth and grain mother: Gaia, Demeter, Ceres—in touch with and encouraging the growth of all things. She is also Venus/Aphrodite: source of love, beauty, luxury, and sensuality. As the imperatrix of creativity, she rules over the imagination. When you embody her energy, relationships come before everything else: the mothering and nurturing relationship to a child, a sexual relationship with a partner, or your creative relationship with an art or craft. Others see you as a graceful and bountiful advocate and patron of the full gamut of the pleasures of life. The negative aspect of Empress consciousness lies in being smothering, jealous, and overwhelming. Generally, she epitomizes mothering, nurturing, and creating.

Ylang-ylang (*Cananga odorata*)[!]—(Water, Venus)

This exquisite flower, whose name means "fragrance of all fragrances," was sacred to the Japanese goddess Amaterasu-o mi-Kami ("heaven radiant great divinity"), highest of the Shinto deities. It is exotic, voluptuous, and erotic but also soothing and relaxing. A true aphrodisiac, it generates feelings of love and creates empathy with others. Dispelling frustration and anger, it stimulates the senses by stimulating the adrenal glands, while relaxing and even sedating tensions and anxiety through regulation of cardiac and respiratory rhythms. By dissolving boundaries, it cures jealousy and makes one receptive to others.

Vanilla (*Vanilla planifolia*)—(Earth/Water, Venus)

Originally from a Mexican orchid worshipped as the manifestation of an Aztec goddess and used in a sacred beverage, vanilla counters melancholy by being a mild stimulant. Its scent is familiar, consoling, and confers a sense of safety and nurturance. It opens us gently to subconscious sensuality and deeply felt emotions, while softening any sense of frustration and anger. It builds confidence and attracts others to us. This is the scent of being enfolded in a mother's arms while cookies bake in the kitchen.

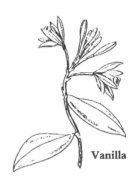
Vanilla

Or, alternately: **Balsam of Peru** (*Myrosperum pereira*), which is actually from Central America.

Rose[4] (*Rosa damascena, centifolia or gallica*)—(Air/Earth, Venus)
Gnostic scriptures say that "the first rose sprouted from the menarchal blood of Psyche, the virgin Soul, when she became enamored of Eros (rose's anagram)."[5] The rose, representing sexual unfolding in all its stages, is for healing of all kinds—for its purity of sexuality touches the soul. Ultimately it promotes a devotion to the eternally creative womb of the Goddess, symbolized in many myths as a rose garden, as was the Muslim paradise called Gulistan after *gul*, the Persian word for rose. It promotes loving relationships, harmonizes all it comes in contact with (including the chakras), and confers beauty. There is no better essence for balanced healing of both men and women, and it elevates all your senses including the spiritual. It expands the aura inclusively, radiates love, and creates an environment of appreciation for aesthetic pleasures. Symbolizing wholeness or completeness, it fills psychic holes. It is the unfolding of love in all its manifestations. (***Palmarosa*** or ***Rose Geranium*** may be substituted.)

4—The Emperor (Fire, Mars, Aries)

The Emperor "rules" the physical world; that is, he makes rules, sets boundaries, names and defines things, and analyzes his domain—which, however,

The Tarot Oils

he did not create. Thus, he administrates and orders what the Empress created. He procreates laws, establishes authority, and energetically directs and focuses the feelings and imagination of the High Priestess and the Empress, initiating new and innovative schemes. Most of all, he seeks immortality—to leave something of himself behind. When you embody the Emperor, you are seen as assertive, positive in outlook, forceful in beliefs, and dynamic about getting things done. You project authority, assume leadership, and feel powerful, but you rely too heavily on what you righteously call reason and the "facts," and you can be dictatorial about insisting that you are right. The Emperor represents fathers and traditional authority figures.

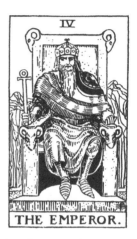

Ginger (*Zingiber officinale*)[!]—(Fire/Water, Mars, Aries/Scorpio)

Ginger is extremely yang, biting, pungent, active, and vibrant. A powerful stimulant, it energizes and strengthens the body and creates sexual desire in men. Ginger instills courage and confidence, promotes aggression and success, and helps you be decisive. While it stimulates the appetite, it also quells nausea (especially motion sickness). Being fiery, it will make you sweat (drink ginger tea before going into a sauna).

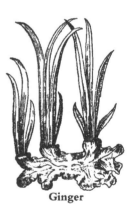

Ginger

Petitgrain (*Citrus bigaradia*)—(Fire, Mars, Aries)

This oil, from the stems and leaves of an orange tree, is surprisingly effective for strengthening your belief in yourself and your abilities. Like other citruses, it counters depression, but also disperses mental confusion by

Essence of Tarot

stimulating the intellect, heightening awareness, and clarifying perceptions. When you feel disappointed or betrayed, it calms anger and reestablishes trust. Its delicacy helps moderate the ego, while still beneficially rectifying your self-regard.

Bay Laurel (*Laurus nobilis* or *Umbellularia californica*)—
(Fire, Sun and Jupiter, Aries/Leo)

Wreaths of laurel were presented to heroes and victors in battle, as well as to poets and athletes, because its "evergreen" nature suggested that their names and deeds would live everlastingly. The word "laureate," therefore, comes from laurel. It indicates recognition and success and signifies the same in business and money magic. Valerie Worwood calls it "distinctive and sexually arrogant." It shields you psychically against another's poisonous or treacherous thoughts, just as the nymph Daphne was protected from Apollo's lecherous intent by being turned into this tree. Sacred to Apollo, Jupiter, Thor, and Gaia (long before the others), it was believed that lightning would never strike it—another sign of high favor. Additionally, it has slight narcotic properties (due to methyl eugenol), which is why the priestesses at Delphi chewed it or inhaled the smoke in order to prophesy. Use for clairvoyance, clear-sightedness, and gaining new perspectives.

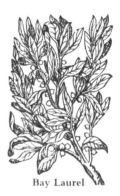

Bay Laurel

5—The Hierophant (Earth, Venus, Taurus)

The Hierophant is a teacher or educational "go-between." Sometimes referred to as the Pontifex ("bridge-builder"), he is society's bridge to traditional values and established knowledge. The Hierophant teaches that which works and has proved itself over time to be reliable, effective, and meaningful. In this card, arcane processes become accessible as expertise is shared. Efforts are focused on problem-solving, emphasizing practical applications of spiritual truths. When you embody the consciousness of the

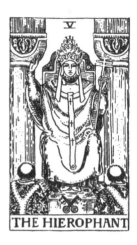

THE HIEROPHANT

Hierophant, others experience you as being able and available to assist them with your expertise and also as being warm and sympathetic. On the other hand, you can be dogmatic and rigid and closed to questions or rebellious attitudes—the important lesson here is to always teach from the heart. You have something important to share, which concerns the manner in which one's earthly actions reverberate through the other planes all the way to Spirit. The Hierophant represents not just teachers but also supervisors, spiritual leaders, and all those who espouse moral, ethical, and spiritual values.

Thyme, White (*Thymus vulgaris*)—(Earth, Venus)
The throat is emphasized in the Hierophant, and thyme is used to soothe it. The word in Greek means courage, and, according to Pliny, the herb will drive off venomous creatures. Today we know that it is twelve times more antiseptic than carbolic acid and will thus help you ward off infection, bacteria, evil traits, or bad values. It stimulates your conscious mind and shuts down your psychic abilities, thus enabling you to take what you've learned from spiritual or intuitive sources and ground it in the material world. With this oil, you can work patiently to develop your resources and absorb new learning more deeply. (Note: *Linalol* is the most gentle form. *Red Thyme* is not recommended for use with children or undiluted.)

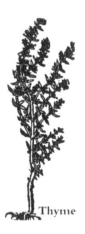
Thyme

Cardamom (*Elettaria cardamomum*)—(Earth/Water, Venus, Taurus)
Interestingly, like thyme, cardamom is also recommended for sore throats, digestion, and—according to Hippocrates—"the bites of venomous crea-

tures." It is a warming spice that stimulates the mind to clear thinking by removing mental fatigue. It is also an aphrodisiac, making men especially feel far more sensual and in touch with their physical bodies. It can help you learn through your senses and open you to teach and guide others from a place of love while remaining consciously clear headed.

Bois de rose (*Rosewood*) (*Aniba rosaeodora*)—(Earth, Venus, Taurus)
The wood is used to make the finest-sounding musical instruments, and the oil from this wood can help you resonate on many levels at once, especially to establish a resonance between student and teacher. It is calming and brings tranquility, but it is not at all sedating, for it stimulates the mind. It banishes fears of abandonment by helping you to feel grounded and secure in yourself and is therefore very constructive whenever you feel emotionally threatened in a new learning situation or when in the presence of an arrogant or pontifical teacher. There is some concern over its use since it only comes from the Amazon rain forest and has become an endangered species.

6—The Lovers (Air, Mercury, Gemini)

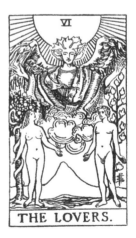

This card is about relationships of all kinds: to family, friends, coworkers, lovers, Spirit, as well as different aspects of ourselves. With its Gemini emphasis, the focus is on communication, and the nudity of the two figures means that we yearn to totally reveal ourselves and be accepted for who we are without hiding anything. When embodying the energy of this card, you may feel split and need to reconcile and balance some duality within yourself, or you may have a conflict between devoting yourself to another or to the urgings of your higher self. What you learned

The Tarot Oils

in the previous card is challenged, so now you need to discriminate between choices. When immersed in the Lovers, people see you as a dual soul, advocating differing points of view until a single image emerges that can encompass them all. Always there is the need to relate—to exchange thoughts and opinions through shared symbols and experience. The Lovers card represents the freedom of choice to be in whatever kind of relationship, whether within ourselves or to others, that we truly want.

Lavender (*Lavandula officinalis, L. vera, L, angustifolia*)—(Air, Mercury and Venus, Gemini/Libra)
The word comes from the Latin *lavandus* meaning "to be washed." Lavender cleanses you of old karmic patterns and emotional conflicts so that you can make choices based on the present. It promotes balance in relationships and helps you to establish that all-important relationship with your higher self—thus it is excellent for meditation and trance channeling. Traditionally it raises spirits, facilitates inner communication, and induces peace and tranquility by dispelling nervousness and depression. It stimulates and regenerates the nervous system and relaxes you when communicating with others. It soothes headaches, and helps with insomnia and irritability. Aromatherapist Kathi Keville finds that using the scent of this gentle oil during childbirth helps to establish first bonds between the parents and child.[6] In dream symbolism, it signifies a reunion. *Lavandin* or *Spike* may also be used.

Geranium (*Pelargonium graveolens, P. odorantissimum*)—(Air, Water, Venus)
This plant tends to excite happiness and harmony in relationships. Relieving stress, it makes you content and predisposed to tenderness and good humor with others. It helps balance aggressive and passive tendencies. According to author Monika Jünemann, it enhances the flow of conversation and facilitates the course of negotiations. Balancing the adrenals and hormones, it also regulates blood pressure, as well as the pressures within a relationship. Although calming anxieties and apprehensions, it is uplifting—stimulating the psyche/soul.

Peppermint (*Mentha piperita*)[!]—(Air, Mercury, Gemini)
Much like Gemini, peppermint favors dual actions: it stimulates the conscious mind while it calms the nerves, and it rapidly alternates cooling and heating actions—but in excess, it can turn from a refreshing sensation to a burning one. When Pluto tried to seduce the naiad Mintha, his wife Queen Persephone transformed her into a low-growing plant but decreed that the more it was walked on the sweeter it would smell. Peppermint represents hidden gifts and beauty that increase your conscious awareness and energy. It also helps with indigestion and headaches. It clears breathing as well as communications and refreshes mental functions. Luckily it also repels pests, so that when working with Lovers energy, you don't have to worry about getting into annoying relationships. A little goes a long way.

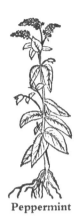
Peppermint

7—The Chariot (Water, Moon, Cancer)

The Chariot is aggressive and forceful, more so than you would imagine for a card associated with Cancer—although remember that it is a cardinal sign. For this reason, Aleister Crowley called it "Mars in Cancer," which can be characterized as a warrior for a cause or the protector of the home. It is also about self-mastery, about evolving an identity keyed to an inner guiding principle. You are called on to develop an ego structure that will direct you toward your goals while keeping your instincts and emotions firmly under control. When you embody the Chariot, others see an aggressive, outgoing person who wants victory, progress, and achievement at almost any cost, but they may not recognize the vulnerable emotional nature that seeks to tear you apart. You need firm and stable roots to feel secure and

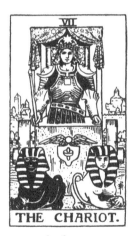

The Tarot Oils

nurtured, because otherwise you tend to act precipitously, riding roughshod over the very things for which you search. The Chariot represents the quest for individuation. It tests your maturity.

Coriander (*Coriandrum sativum*)—(Fire/Water, Mars, Scorpio)

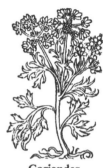
Coriander

Coriander is a gentle stimulant that urges you into action. It focuses your concentration on activities rather than on more sedate endeavors and relieves stress and anxiety—especially that arising from shock or fear. It encourages you to move and quickens your native ingeniousness—and so speeds your progress toward a goal. Its aphrodisiac qualities are provocative and revivifying, so use it when you feel a lag in your energy.

Carrot (*Daucus carota*)—(Fire/Water, Sun and Mars, Cancer)

To the Greeks, this was an aphrodisiac called Philtron. The 16th-century botanical alchemist Leonhardt Thurneisserus described it as both Sun and Mars in Cancer, which was borne out by electrical experiments in 1927 that found the carrot "very excitable." According to author Patricia Davis, it "strengthens inner vision, enabling the user to perceive the highest truth at times of doubt or confusion." Thus the light of the star on the Charioteer's crown can be a clear guide, overriding the confusion of the opposing sphinxes or horses. Carrot also removes energy blocks.

Labdanum (*Cistus ladanifer*)—(Water, Moon, Cancer/Scorpio)

This gum from the European rock rose was thought erroneously to come from a shellfish—thus its traditional association with Cancer because of the symbolism of the crab. Used in Babylonia for the oldest-known temple incense, it heralded their new year while the story of "En Elish" was read, and it was called the "victory of the Lord." Therefore it is most appropriate for a card that is also called "Victory." It instills courage and a willingness to risk yourself to help others by overcoming doubt and fright.

Chamomile (Roman) (*Anthemis nobilis, A. mixta*)—(Water, Moon, Cancer)
Chamomile brings you the remarkable serenity of the moon, which rules Cancer. It induces sleep, peacefulness, and meditation. Chamomile relieves tension and dispels anger and irritation. It can even heal you after too much sun. Clearing away past emotional concerns, it opens the pathways for intuitive channeling of your deepest knowledge from within to help you find your way.

8—Strength (Fire, Sun, Leo)

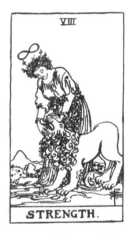

Strength signifies accepting your instincts and your own inner nature so as to work in harmony with that energy. You are a part of nature, but your will does not have to be at odds with your natural desires. Personal integrity and a strong willpower come from valuing your feelings rather than trying to strangle them, including having respect for your rage and anger. Your intellect and will, though, can direct these urges into appropriate channels of expression. Like an enchantress, you tame raw energy and transform it into the strength to succeed. When you embody Strength, others see you as having a passion for life, the courage to engage your heart to its fullest, and the power to express your unique and vital abilities. Strength represents unity of mind and heart, of body and soul. Like Leo, its power comes from the heart.

Rosemary (*Rosemarinus officinalis*)[!]—(Fire, Sun, Leo)
Rosemary symbolizes love and remembrance and is sacred to friendship. It was used in both bridal wreaths and students' head wreaths, because it

The Tarot Oils

forges strong links among friends, lovers, ideas and knowledge, the past and present, ancestors and descendants, and body and soul. Its ability to drive away evil spirits and make fearsome animals timid is perfect for approaching and calming the wild beast within. It is associated with wisdom, love, and loyalty. It is said that where rosemary flourishes, the mistress (Goddess) rules, and its name comes from *ros marinus*, "dew of the sea," because it grows best next to the ocean depths of the Great Mother. It refreshes and awakens by warming and stimulating the circulation of blood through the

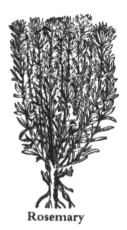

Rosemary

heart; therefore use it in the morning to help get you going. It has long been considered a psychic protector, especially against malevolent magic. It clears the mind, provokes philosophical thinking and brings forth creativity. Generous of spirit, it quickens all the senses by lifting exhaustion and lethargy. Use it to help you learn who you are and how to be strong in yourself.

Juniper (Juniperus communis)—(Fire, Sun, Leo)

The red berries of the juniper, sacred to Inanna and Ishtar, have been burned by many peoples for spiritual purification and to keep evil spirits away. Ancient Tibetan shamans used them in the *Sang Cho* or "smoke offering." The juniper and its attendant elves and fairies guard homes and animals, warding off negativity, usually by creating some kind of distraction. Barbara Walker quotes a children's rhyme that goes: "Do not betray what the juniper bush has to protect."[7] Used for general healing, it detoxifies the body by its action as a diuretic and blood purifier. For inner strength, it helps you hold onto your highest ideals, while ridding you of excess things, including unwanted emotional attachments. It is a psychic stimulant and aid to meditation and has been used for both love potions and for attack—especially as it attacks and cleanses psychic uncleanliness. As a flavoring in gin, it helps to raise other kinds of spirits.

Neroli (*Citrus aurantium bigarade*)—(Fire, Sun, Leo)

This is specifically from the orange blossom, rather than any other part of the plant. Although this is a solar energy, it is also intensely female. Valerie Worwood recommends neroli oil for facing emotional fear. "It calms highly charged emotional states and redirects the energies." Although a powerful antidepressant and good for insomnia, it is also stimulating, energetic, and confidence-building. It makes you self-aware and benefits the heart. It enhances creativity by releasing emotional tension so that ideas flow smoothly. The plant is used in wedding rituals because the white blossom represents purity (like the white maiden), while the fruit represents fertility, and both can appear on a tree at one time. It promises mutual sexual satisfaction. It creates links between your lower and higher selves, and, according to author Gurudas, it enables you to directly communicate with possessing entities or your obsessions. In other words, it calms the savage beast and your emotional fears and rampages so that you can establish communications and healing links.

Or, alternately: *Orange* (*Citrus aurantium*). Orange oil comes from the peel rather than the blossom. According to Barbara Walker, in European witchcraft it represented the heart. Orange does not reach the same spiritual heights as neroli but creates a joyous, lively outlook by dispersing fear of the unknown and releasing obsessions. Its ability to transform depression into peace nourishes the soul and can help us to relax into sleep.

9—The Hermit (Earth, Mercury, Virgo)

The Hermit deals with solitude and introspection and is about learning through self-reflection. It is also about how you serve others through the knowledge you have gained. Thus the Hermit figure, called the "way shower," as he sheds his light for others to follow, offers a clear perspective from the mountain peak of pure abstract thought. The star that lights the way is that which appeared on the helmet of the Charioteer: a goal you now have the wisdom to handle. The

The Tarot Oils

card suggests prudence and perfectionism but also independence. When you embody the Hermit, others see you as a loner but also as a role model of personal integrity. Your experience suggests maturity and self-sufficiency, and you are perceived as purposeful but can also seem impersonal, overly cautious, and even prudish. Besides representing the wise old man, the Hermit on a more esoteric level is the wise old woman, Hecate, especially in her form as Queen Persephone who guides souls into the underworld in winter and back to rebirth in spring.

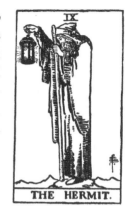

Sage (*Salvia officinalis*)[!!]—(Earth/Air, Mercury, Jupiter)
The word sage comes from the Latin root *sap*—meaning "taste," hence judgement and wisdom—implying that wisdom comes from the senses. The Latin plant name, *salvia*, means "whole or healthy." Therefore the Hermit maintains health by using the senses wisely. Because in magic the herb corresponds to money, we have the result that the sage is "healthy, wealthy, and wise." An Arabic saying declares that sage renders men immortal: "How shall a man die who has sage in his garden?" This oil is for clarity in thinking and in speaking your intentions. Its salutary qualities fortify you for the spiritual quest within yourself, yet, as Gurudas points out, keeps you from becoming a religious fanatic. It stimulates the brain, memory, liver, and spiritual opening and is thought to promote longevity.

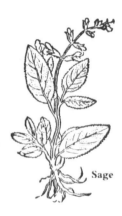

Wintergreen (*Gaultheria procumbens*) or *Birch* (*Betula lenta*)[!]—(Earth, Mercury, Virgo)
"Oil of wintergreen" from a small shrub is almost identical to that of the sweet birch tree, as they both are mostly methyl salicylate (used to flavor

Essence of Tarot

cola and root beer). The scent sharpens the senses and stimulates the mind, being reminiscent of a high mountain lake. Witches were thought to fly on broomsticks of birch, representing Hecate traveling to a gathering of wise women. It is a penetrating body rub, extremely good for muscle or joint pain, but should be highly diluted or it will irritate the skin. A symbol of grace and humbleness, it was thought that hanging birch branches indoors would protect the home. Use it for wisdom journeys.

Caraway (*Carum Carvi*)—(Air/Earth, Mercury, Virgo)
Caraway is also reminiscent of flying away. Like most of the herbs of the Umbelliferae family, it is refreshing to the conscious mind, enhancing alertness, strengthening memory, and promoting clear communications. It also revitalizes the physical body. Encouraging the qualities of giving and receiving, it thus attracts others. It stimulates the digestion and lymphatic system.

Caraway

Narcissus (*Narcissus* spp.)[!]—(Earth, Mercury, Virgo)
Narcissus comes from the Greek *narkao*, meaning "to be numb," because the bulb can cause paralysis and even death. Sophocles named it "the garland of the great infernal goddess, because they that are departed and dulled with death, should worthily be crowned with a numbing flower." Although difficult to find, it belongs here (perhaps use the flower essence) because its myth is especially significant for the Hermit card.

The narcissus flower was grown by Gaia so that its fragrance would lure the maiden Persephone to sleep in a place where the god of the underworld, Pluto, could abduct her. Thus it has been called a flower of deceit. Esoterically this card represents Persephone traveling in and out of the underworld in her manifestation as Hecate, the Crone. As the first flower to bloom in the spring, it represents the rebirth of Persephone into the world. Because of its association with the youth who stared at himself in a reflecting pool until he was turned into the flower, it represents self-contemplation, introversion, and self-sufficiency.

The Tarot Oils

The Furies wore narcissus flowers among their tangled locks to keep them so stupefied they could do no harm to others, and a Sufi saying goes, "Smell a narcissus, even if only once a day or once a week or once a month or once a year or once a lifetime. For verily in the heart of man there is the seed of insanity, leprosy, and leukoderma. And the scent of narcissus drives them away."[8] It brings calm and deep relaxation that allows one to descend deeply into the hidden and often frightening aspects of the psyche. There you can confront your deepest fears and "own" the rejected parts of yourself so as to bring them into the light of consciousness and thus become whole.

10—The Wheel of Fortune (Fire/Water, Jupiter)

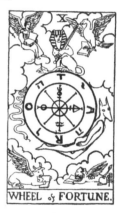

The Wheel of Fortune is concerned with change, movement, expansion, and opportunity. It allows you to obtain a centralized view of the whole—a sort of philosophical perspective—but sometimes it seems as though you are just along for the ride, especially if you find yourself thrust onto the periphery of the wheel, hanging on for dear life. This card is about how your fate unravels as the seasons change and how you change with them. It often brings rewards and recognition for things you've completed. When you embody the Wheel, you seem to take continual risks as you reach for each new opportunity and meet every challenge, and yet Lady Luck seems to help you land on your feet. On the other hand, you can appear to be impatient and even superficial, broad and scattered rather than having precision and depth. The Wheel of Fortune represents changing times, the ups and downs of your experience, and the opportunity to perceive reoccurring cycles and patterns.

Cedar (*Cedrus* spp., esp. *C. atlantica*)[!]—(Fire, Jupiter)
Cedar represents power and longevity, strength and beauty. The Bible says, "the righteous . . . shall grow like a cedar in Lebanon" (Psalms 92:12). Because it repels insects, it has been used in the preservation and dissemination of books, words, and, therefore, philosophies, yet it is a mild sedative, relaxing the analytical mind. Cleansing and protecting, it promotes spiritual energy and calms and deepens focus for ceremony. It enhances honor, wealth, and dignity. Just as its astringent qualities cut through mucus and catarrh, so it can cut through mental muck and relieve tension. It promotes clarity of thought that moves to the center of an issue, rather than remaining peripheral. (**American Cedar** can be substituted, which is really from the *Juniperus* species.)

Nutmeg (*Myristica fragrans*)[!]—(Fire, Jupiter, Sagittarius)
This oil is for prosperity and for bringing money and luck into your life. Its optimism fights depression and tiredness, overcoming mental fatigue, confusion, and lethargy. Its volatility promotes higher thought, but it can also be warm and seductive. Being narcotic, it can bring intense and colorful dreams or cause headaches. Be careful, because it can raise you up only to cast you down if you overindulge in it. Nutmeg oil is one of the major ingredients in a perfume called frangipani, created by a 16th-century Italian noblewoman and not to be confused with the Hawaiian plumeria flower that is also called frangipani. The 16th-century recipe is reportedly one of the few aphrodisiacs used by women for their own enjoyment.

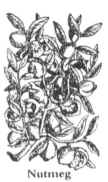

Nutmeg

Clove (*Syzygium aromaticum*)—(Fire, Jupiter, Sagittarius)
Clove is a powerful germicide and the source of eugenol, used in dentistry. It eases pain and destroys parasites. Thus it fortifies you during uncomfortable

changes and helps with the pain of letting go of situations that no longer serve your growth. An energy booster, it stimulates the brain and brings up old memories and reoccurring patterns so you can see them in a new light. It is protective as well as attractive, drawing to you only those things on which you focus your will. You can use it with visualization and affirmation to painlessly create the kinds of changes you want.

Saffron (Crocus sativum)—(Fire, Jupiter, Leo/Sagittarius)
This is an expensive oil, but it well represents both material prosperity and spiritual achievement. At one time it set the standard for what was rare and expensive. Used by the Persians and Greeks to raise the wind and resurrect the dead, its aphrodisiac power could cause women to swoon and was thus considered equal to gold in causing their corruption. In small amounts it "quickens the senses, makes merry, shakes off drowsiness," said the herbalist Gerard, but too much creates disaster: Jason and Medea used it for their death-dealing witch brews. It was sacred in Crete and was used throughout the ancient world to dye priestly robes with the golden saffron color signifying the perfection of divinity. In moderation, it strengthens the soul, dispels melancholy, spurs vitality, and develops spiritual values. In excess, it makes one mad with desire and corrupts the soul. The winds of change blow powerfully and suddenly with saffron.

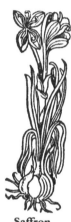

Saffron

11—Justice (Air, Venus, Libra)

Justice is the card of balance, agreements, negotiations, and decisions. But at a deeper level, it is about being true to yourself and your own nature, or else none of your agreements with others will be truly fair and just. Justice shows how you balance your needs with those of another and how you can live with the consequences of the decisions you make. You learn to weigh the pros and cons, to analyze and evaluate the factors, to list the facts, and make value judgements about whether something is good or bad—but you must be flexible enough to make adjustments for your underlying feelings and to honor your personal truth. When you embody Justice, others see you as being fair and morally upright, seeing both sides of the issue, yet standing firm and making clear decisions once the truth is known. Justice represents taking the responsibility to adjust the imbalances in your life.

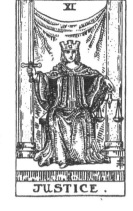

Myrtle (*Myrtus communis*)—(Air, Venus, Libra)
Myrtle, coming from a word that means "sea goddess" and "female genitals" and related to the Sumerian *Marienna*, meaning "high fruitful mother of heaven," has a rich and varied mythology. In the Garden of Eden it was chief of the scented trees, and when Adam and Eve were expelled from paradise, they were allowed to take the most fragrant plant with them. Coming as it does from paradise, it is one of the "angelic" energies, symbolizing promise, bounty, and atonement for sins. It was the sacred plant of

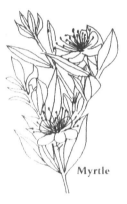

the goddess Aphrodite, in which she sought refuge after being born naked in the foam of the sea. It is used as an amulet against shipwreck, and therefore protects you through life transitions and emotional upheavals.

Good for all lung conditions, it cleanses the inner being by dissolving disharmony. Like the two-edged sword indicating the power of life and death, it also can signify endings—especially the karmic ending of an old cycle. It represented the last month of the old king's reign, while the wild olive represented the first month of the next king's reign. Myrtle wands were used for communication with the dead. It was the myrtle nymphs, as prophetesses, who taught the children of Cyrene and Apollo to cultivate the olive, for myrtle signified the end of an epoch and was carried by victors to mark their colonization and cultivation of a land. Aphrodite turned her priestess Myrene into the plant so that she should be green throughout the year, and it is therefore also an emblem of the immortality of love and respect. Its use to crown poets and athletes (called an *ovation*, inferior to a *triumph*) marked their ever-green fame.

Perhaps the heart of these stories arises from the warrior priestesses of the goddess Myrine on Lemnos, who were lovingly immortalized as namesakes of this plant after their culture was overcome by the patriarchal Greeks. This plant secretly kept the memory of matriarchal rulership alive, indicated by the fact that it brought luck but could only be planted by a woman. It represents pride and the preservation of love, thus well represents Justice's injunction that to be fair and just, you must first be "true to yourself."

Palmarosa (*Cymbopogon martinii*)—(Air, Venus, Libra)
This light sweet oil is related to lemongrass, but its rose scent makes it effective for love magic. It helps clarify your thoughts about partnerships (and contractual agreements) and sharpens the senses. It is valuable for skin healing and cellular regeneration and transmutes pathogenic intestinal flora into healthy ones. Especially good against anorexia, it allows you to be loving to yourself instead of harshly judgmental.

Spearmint (*Mentha spicata*)—(Air, Mercury, Libra)
Spearmint is called "menthe de Notre Dame." Its stimulant action is more gentle than peppermint, yet it still provides clarity in decision-making and promotes personal integrity and wisdom. It is good for balancing your needs with those of another and offers hospitality and partnership. On the other hand, Demeter turned a man into a lizard who laughed because she gulped down barley water flavored with mint, so it can also indicate swift retribution for perceived transgressions.

12—The Hanged Man (Water, Neptune)

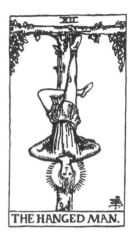

The Hanged Man depicts the consciousness of devotion, egolessness, and sacrifice. It may indicate that you feel powerless in the face of injustice or powerless to escape your fate, obsessions, or personal situation. You need to suspend all judgements and surrender to a higher power, trusting in a better outcome than you could create by yourself. You may be completely wrapped up in an inner world or entranced by the astral plane. You may be devoted to another—a spiritual leader or personal relationship—or hung up in some sort of addiction. You may be lost in the creative process, unaware of the passage of time or sense of self. When you embody the Hanged Man, others see you as sensitive, imaginative, idealistic, or perhaps baffled and confused—but anyway, not very realistic. You may seem to be drifting or humbly waiting for something to happen, rather than initiating action. This card represents the mystic, the shaman, and the dreamer—who, in recognizing the paradoxes and mysteries of life, perceive experience from a different, sometimes opposite, perspective from the rest of the world.

Mugwort (*Artemisia vulgaris*)[!!]—(Water, Moon and Neptune, Pisces)
From the earliest times, this silver plant that glows in the moonlight has been associated with magic and witchcraft. In the Middle Ages, it was used to anoint magic mirrors and crystals for crystal gazing and to see spirits or events at a distance (scrying). As it always turns to the north, it was thought to be magnetically influenced. Hung above the door (especially at Midsummer), it warded off lightning and the devil. Although it promotes dreams, visions, and astral travel, it does not bring sleep, for it keeps the journeyer from becoming weary. Used in purification ceremonies, it balances psychic

"moon forces," opens the intuition and the subconscious, and increases all flows. Thus it is a woman's plant, treating delayed menstruation. Compressed, it is used for moxibustion in acupuncture to stimulate blocked energies.

Take extreme care when using essential oil of mugwort. This oil should never be used corporeally without expert supervision. Topical use is potentially dangerous. Pregnant women or those who are seeking to conceive should avoid this oil, as it may cause uterine contractions. Essential oil of mugwort must *never* be consumed or otherwise taken internally, as it is potentially highly toxic in this form. However, tea made from dried mugwort *leaves*—not the essential oil!—may be safe to drink, although, again, not for the pregnant or those who are seeking to conceive.

Spikenard (*Nardostachys jatamansi*)—(Water/Earth, Saturn and Neptune)
Greatly esteemed by the Egyptians, Romans, and Hebrews, it is said to comfort the heart. As mentioned earlier, it was used by Mary Magdalene, a temple priestess of the goddess Astarte (patron saint of perfumes), in the sacred ritual of Chrism, marking Jesus as the "chosen one" and giving him the strength for his coming task. According to Patricia Davis, spikenard intensifies the feeling of devotion towards the deity or a spiritual teacher. Valerian, which is related, comes from a word meaning "strong," and therefore it gives strength and comfort when working with disenfranchised people and seemingly hopeless causes. Spikenard is for those who deeply empathize with the suffering of others. Used as a nerve tonic, it helps you relax and sleep, and it is good for migraine sufferers. North American Indians used it as a smudge in the belief that it cured insanity.

Myrrh (*Commiphora myrrha*)[!]—(Water, Moon, Saturn and Neptune, Pisces)
The name means "bitter tears," being related to both *mar* (ocean) and *mari* (bitter), and signifies a mother's sorrow. It is for healing wounds, representing the wounded-healer archetype, and for mystical understanding. Like mugwort, it opens the womb and promotes menses, which is perhaps why it says in the Bible that women to be married were purified for "six months with oil of

myrrh" (Esther 2:12). Adonis (a sacrificed god whose story can be equated with that of Tammuz and Ishtar, and Jesus and Mary) was born to a woman named Myrrha, who was turned into a myrrh tree for incest with her father. The tree bark burst after ten month's gestation to give birth to Adonis. The tear-like resin of myrrh that oozes from the bark represents the tears of Myrrha at the death of her son and was ritually burned at the festival of Adonis. Myrrh prefigured Christ's sacrifice at his birth and was given to him when he hung on the cross. Considered mysterious and seductive, it was a major ingredient in the Egyptian *Kyphi*, burned at sunset when Ra descended into the underworld, and in the consecration oil of the Hebrews.

13—Death (Water, Mars and Pluto, Scorpio)

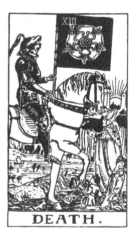

Death signifies an aggressive surge toward creative life-energy, which may manifest as clearing the way for growth to take place. It represents destruction in preparation for renewal, or dismemberment so that regeneration can take place. It is the rich, decayed loam of compost that feeds new growth. Knowing that you will someday die, hating death becomes equivalent to hating life. When you embody the energy of this card, others see in you an intensity and depth of passion that is almost frightening. You don't take anything lightly, and you eliminate everything not necessary to your essential purpose. You peel back the layers of robes and skin, of beauty and wealth, of power and ambition—to find what really supports you. Death represents letting go of your personal will and releasing outgrown or outmoded forms.

Cypress (*Cupressus sempervirens*)—(Water, Venus and Pluto, Libra/Scorpio)
The Cypress will not grow again once cut, so it signified the permanency of death, yet its name means "ever-living." Supposedly it was named after

Cyparissus, who was turned into a cypress so that he could mourn his playmate, a stag whom he had been tricked into killing—for the cypress tree shaded the pool of Lethe, or "forgetfulness," in the underworld. Planted in cemeteries as an ancient symbol of comfort and solace, it is used for soothing transitions of all kinds, particularly the loss of friends and loved ones or the endings of relationships. It eases losses and promotes healing through its sedative action. Helpful in transitions, Patricia Davis recommends it for career changes, moving from home, and for major spiritual decisions. Cypress was sacred on the isle of Cyprus, where it was dedicated to Aphrodite, the love goddess born of foam, sperm, and moisture. Thus, acting through the ovaries, cypress is helpful in menopause and for menstrual disorders. It is especially symbolic of feminine maturity and strength and is of great use in menopause rituals. Valerie Worwood says it eases sadness, yet is direct and outspoken, helping us to stand up for ourselves with enigmatic pride. It was part of an Old Testament tree riddle whose answer was Chokmah, the source of wisdom, suggesting that sadness and grief bring wisdom.

Rue (*Ruta graveolens*)[!!!]—(Fire, Mars, Aries/Scorpio)
As is appropriate to the Death card, rue is one of the most toxic of available essential oils. It should be used with great care and greatly diluted (never more than one drop per ¼ to ½ ounce of carrier oil and *never* internally. From the Greek word *reuo*, it means "to be set free" and was believed to cure illness or poisoning. The Greeks made an anointing oil using rue juice and dew from the moonwort (*Lunaria*), placing it on the head of a person for protection. As a potent antimagical herb, it is used for uncrossing hexes and for psychic self-defense (by closing down your psychic receptivity). Scott Cunningham recommends it for easing the pain of broken relationships and lessening the ache of unreciprocated love. It calms raging emotions. Priests in the Catholic Church sprayed holy water around the church by dipping a spring of rue in consecrated water then shaking it.

Since many essential oil suppliers will not even offer rue, **Valerian** (*Valerian officinalis*) may be substituted. It is similar in effect to spikenard as described under The Hanged Man.

Cumin (*Cuminum cyminum*), which is related to Mars, may also be substituted. It is good for lymphatic conditions and poor circulation and, as Scott Cunningham points out, has an odor strong enough to melt cosmetics (and metaphorically to melt flesh from bone). Use it to protect your home. As a remedy against indigestion and constipation, it helps in all elimination processes.

Opoponax (*Commiphora erythraea*)—(Water, Pluto, Scorpio)
Opoponax, also called bisabol or bdellium, is a gum related to myrrh but darker—like spicy wine—and more intense. Arctander thought its "vegetable-soup-like, slightly animal-sweet odor" was "entirely different from the medicinal-sharp freshness" of myrrh. Aleister Crowley, to whom it represented the fiery part of water, said it contained the "overpowering richness of the deliciously abominable," while the name itself means "all-healing vegetable juice." It is a major ingredient of incense in China. Like myrrh, it represents release from the physical.

14—Temperance (Fire, Jupiter, Sagittarius)

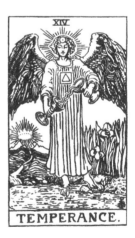

The card Temperance signifies rebirth and renewal after the letting-go of the previous card. Temperance refers to having compassion for mistakes and using your ability to heal yourself by correcting imbalances and reconciling opposing beliefs. It turns stress into creative challenge. You learn to creatively combine contrary forces into new entities. Temperance represents humanism and idealism—and your own attempts to find solutions, bridge gaps, and catalyze change. When you embody Temperance, others see you as manifesting your own highest self, or as your guardian angel. You affirm wholeness, beauty, strength, and the ability to accomplish whatever you desire. In turn, you urge others to try and try again, demonstrating how guilt and errors can actually be blessings. As a networker and wholistic healer, you make connections and associations, and by paying attention to timing and temperature, you can adjust and redistribute energy in order that things function at their best. Temperance represents the alchemist, the aromatherapist, and your own deepest guidance.

Hyssop (*Hyssopus officinalis*)[!!]—(Fire, Jupiter, Sagittarius)
A plant of the winter solstice, and therefore rebirth, hyssop was used by the Egyptians and the Hebrews to sweep out their temples for cleansing and purification. Its Hebrew name, *azob*, means "holy herb," and with it you can acknowledge and then release guilt. As Psalm 51:7 directs, "Purge me with hyssop, and I shall be clean: wash me, and I shall be whiter than snow." Therefore, use it in baths and lustrations as a preparation for serious rituals (although not if pregnant or epileptic). It quickly clears the mind of psychological debris, producing a feeling of alertness and clarity. It can be part of a balancing tonic (an anointing elixir or massage oil) that regulates blood pressure, as well as for stimulation and relaxation, aggressiveness and sedation. A symbol for baptism and forgiveness of sins, it uplifts, rejuvenates, gives wings to your spirits without letting you lose touch with reality. It cleanses the chest and clears the respiratory tract. In traditional magic, it assures faithfulness of friends and lovers, financial success, purification, and protection during exorcism.

Bergamot (*Citrus bergamia*)[!]—(Fire/Air, Sun and Jupiter, Sagittarius)
Bergamot, a kind of orange, is a softly radiant oil. It heals by opening your heart to joy, especially when you are experiencing grief. It is soothing and uplifting. It helps you to sleep, yet it is mentally stimulating and refreshing to the spirit. Balancing the activity of the hypothalamus, it helps you maintain the appropriate temperature and temperament, and it is especially good for eating disorders. Bergamot promotes self-assurance and self-confidence by enhancing your sense of personal beauty and individual distinction. It is an animating antidepressant, yet it mellows and cools excessive heat. It helps you be clear about your objectives, so is good for

traveling and when undertaking problem-solving tasks. However, its solar quality actually increases photosensitivity, so purchase a bergaptene-free version if you wish to apply it to your body.

Angelica (*Angelica archangelica*)—(Fire, Sun, Sagittarius)
This herb has a fiery temperament and reaches toward the heavens, yet it is solidly grounded with strong roots (it is sometimes called "root of the Holy Ghost") and therefore strengthens the spirit. It is called angelica because it facilitates contact with angelic energies and alignment with the higher self. It helps you see problems clearly, especially from new perspectives, and helps you decide about new directions to take. It bolsters you when you are feeling too timid, weak, or lacking in perseverance to continue. It treats imbalances in the menstrual cycle, blood cells and circulation, and in psychological states by bonding different parts of the personality. Use it for balance, guidance, to overcome difficulties, and in altered-states work (hypnotherapy, channeling, etc.) for protection and insight into the root of any problem. (Because the oil is expensive, and it is the subtle energies you will want to contact, you can use the flower essence instead.)

15—The Devil (Earth, Saturn, Capricorn)

The Devil is about fear. You may, upon looking at the card, either think that you've done something "bad" (guilt) or that something nasty is about to happen. Fears contain tremendous energy that is repressed and blocked from natural creative expression, building up into monstrous images of abusive power that manifest as projected evil in others (dictators or scapegoats), germs and viruses, nightmares, and personal guilt. It may indicate that you are trespassing on social or sexual taboos—and that you may respond with deceit, obsession, manipulation, and pride—or see these things all around you. This card refers to ambition and to playing the games required in the hard world of material possessions and one-upmanship.

The Tarot Oils

The Devil energy concerns constriction and the limitations that external forces seem to impose on you. Underneath all of this is a failure to love, with the resulting sense of isolation and separateness. On the other hand, the Devil can represent the Horned God and rampant sexuality. When you embody the Devil, others see you either as manipulative and imposing or as devilishly playful: taunting, challenging, stirring up the things no one wants to look at. The key to this card is keeping a sense of humor and recognizing the creative energy available here. The Devil represents the monster at the threshold, guarding a treasure of great worth.

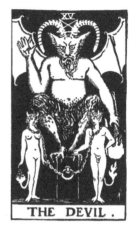

Clary Sage (*Salvia sclarea*)[!!]—(Earth/Air, Saturn and Mercury, Capricorn)
Clary sage, a very useful oil, is best known for dealing with paranoia and panic—coming from Pan, a less frightening name for the devil. It brings euphoria and even intoxication, emphasizing the "mirthful" quality of the archetype. Its ability to remedy melancholy helps you to ground yourself, to relax and smile, so use it for depression and facing your fears. With its ability to awaken curiosity, clarify, and embolden, its use leads to self-realization and self-knowledge. Being warm and seductive, it stimulates sexual response, especially in women, and can induce erotic dreams, helping you to break through sexual repression and guilt. It is especially good for midlife crises and menopausal hot flashes. (Although given warning marks, it is actually quite safe except during pregnancy; or when mixed with alcohol intake, as the combination can then produce nightmares and headaches.)

Patchouli (*Pogostemon cablin, P. patchouli*) [!]—(Earth, Venus and Saturn, Taurus/Capricorn)
This dark, earthy, almost animal-like oil is richly scented but at times too voluptuous or forceful; some people even find it repellent. It helps

you deal with anxiety and self-doubt. Arousing sexuality, it suggests an intense union that dissolves boundaries and is used in Tantric practices. In any case, it releases anxieties about sexuality. Although it awakens a desire for the unconventional, it also grounds your stirred energies and makes you aware of your body. It reveals your obsessions by reaching deep into your emotions, elevates depression, and puts things into perspective. Because it improves with aging or drying, it prolongs beauty in maturity and is rejuvenating in that it regenerates skin cells. It repels moths. Traditionally it has been used in money magic to bring financial and business success.

16—The Tower (Fire, Mars)

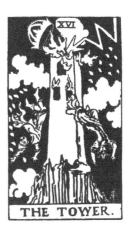

The Tower concerns breakthroughs and breakdowns: mental, physical, and spiritual. It shatters whatever has become rigid and unyielding and throws you out of limiting situations. When under its influence, you may lose control and can explode or blow up in anger. Energies that have been repressed for too long are released. It leads to aggressive action, arguments, and even violence. On the other hand, the lightning represents insights from the higher self that open you to new possibilities, and the flames are your drive to take action. When you embody the Tower, others may see you as angry and destructive or as dynamic, assertive, and exciting. You clear out debris, burn through obstructions, cleanse and renovate. The Tower symbolizes the ejaculatory force of the creative impulse.

Black Pepper (*Piper nigrum*)—(Fire, Mars, Aries)
Black pepper, although not as hot and sharp as the spice itself, can stimulate your mind and body into action. It is excellent for mental alertness

The Tarot Oils

and concentration and can keep you awake during meditations. It bolsters courage, sharpens your self-defensive abilities, and builds your ability to confront difficult or dangerous situations. Its heat remedies physical and emotional cold. A stimulating aphrodisiac, it adds stamina and strength to the physical act. It also removes blocks to energy movement between the chakras by seeking out hidden anger and frustration.

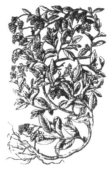

Black Pepper

Pine (*Pinus* spp.)—(Air, Mars, Aries/Scorpio)
The pine hungers for light and awakens the life spirit. Very individualistic, it suggests longevity and loneliness. It is sacred to Dionysus and to Pan because of its affinity with grapes, which grow where it grows; also, pine resin was used to conserve and refine wine. The pinecone is a symbol of fertility and activates the pineal gland, which is named after it. It is said that upon the death of Attis (a vegetation god of sacrifice), he changed into a pine, just as Osiris was shown enclosed in a pine at his shrine at Denderah. Like the Tower, pine signifies the male erection. The oil is cleansing, exhilarating, and speeds recuperation from illness, giving a will to live, courage, and strength. It promotes feelings of energy and well-being and intensifies breathing and blood circulation, which supports detoxification processes. Use it as a male stimulant to treat impotency or disinterest or to excite love in the face of adversity. Used for winter purifications, it repels negative energies while increasing bioelectrical energy. In rituals, it is used for invoking Pan.

Sassafras (*Sassafras albidum*)[!!]—(Fire, Mars, Aries)
A general tonic, sassafras deals with all kinds of eruptions, including those on the skin. In saunas, it treats general weakness and mental problems and fights exhaustion. Because it clears the eyes, it can be considered for insight. Its active ingredient, isosafrole, is also found in nutmeg and in the psychedelic drug MDA. Beware, highly toxic sassafras oil should *never* be ingested.

17—The Star (Air, Saturn and Uranus, Aquarius)

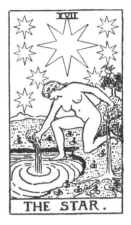

The Star is about self-esteem and a hopeful vision of humanity in an ecologically sound relationship with the planet and the universe, especially important in this period of intense climate change. It offers a sense of deep connection between the stars and the earth, the above and the below. Under the cool night sky, you renew not only your own resources but also the vital structures and balance of the planet. With divine grace, you joyfully and humbly strive to preserve life. You recognize the need for discipline, repetition, and order, which provide a basis for serenity in meditation, yet you have the assurance required to be the "star of the show." When you embody the energy of the Star, others see you as uninhibited and free yet aware of a personal destiny that is also universal. You seem charismatic, free thinking, and innovative. Your commitment to honesty, growth, and to the future is clear. The Star signifies the beauty, order, and interdependency of nature.

Eucalyptus (*Eucalyptus globulus*)—(Air, Mercury and Uranus, Aquarius)
Refreshing and stimulating, eucalyptus is excellent for breathing exercises and for meditation. According to Monika Jünneman, it helps you to experience the transcendental nature of your relationships to others and to the earth. It dispels negative psychic energy, cools fevers, and is good for migraines. It soothes eruptions, which is good after the disruption of the Tower, and protects you from evil and mental anguish. Its purifying action brings peace where there was conflict and disagreement. Increasing intellectual perception, it helps you to see other people's point of view and to learn from your mistakes.

Fir (*Abies balsamea*)—(Air, Saturn, Aquarius)
Fir is grounding, yet it opens energy blocks, elevates emotions, and increases intuition. Sacred to Artemis, it is known as a birth tree and, as *ailm* (its early

name), was the first letter of an early Druid alphabet. It was sacred to the moon goddess Elate (or Pitys), and Pan's satyrs wore fir twigs in their hair in her honor. Like the star in the sky, or the candles lit in its branches at winter solstice, the fir heralded the birth of the sun. As an evergreen, it symbolizes ongoing life and immortality. It increases your contentment, making you feel at home on this planet, while fostering your ability to accept and share love.

Lime (*Citrus aurantifolia*)—(Air, Sun, Aquarius)
Lime is loud and self-assured. A mental stimulant and energy restorer, it impels you into action. It is psychologically opening and freeing. A source of vitamin C and a great healing agent in fevers and infection, it also prevents scurvy (which is how the British sailors came to be called "limeys"). It lends creditability to your principled and high-minded honesty. In Malaysia, the tree is the patron of actors, so will help you shine as the "star" of the show.

Blue (or *German*) *Chamomile* (*Matricaria chamomilla*)—(Air/Water, Uranus, Aquarius)
Just as Roman chamomile and the High Priestess represent Isis veiled, so the blue chamomile and Star goddess represent Isis unveiled—the goddess naked beneath the nighttime sky. *Matricaria* means "mothering," and here the goddess nurtures the cosmos. Containing blue crystals of azulene, blue chamomile is an excellent anti-inflammatory agent. It calms hysteria, hyperactivity, and nervous stress, and it is gentle enough to use with children. Stimulating the

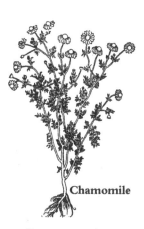
Chamomile

pineal gland, it creates, through meditation, a sense of harmony and organization and helps with the objective assimilation of higher wisdom and linear, academic information. Its objectivity is excellent for those who are oversensitive. It helps you focus on your life path and overcomes any anger, anxiety, or bitterness that gets in the way of speaking your truth.

18—The Moon (Water, Jupiter and Neptune, Pisces)

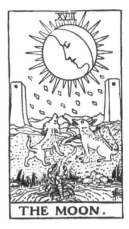

The Moon card is about spiritual evolution. Its images, however, depict the fears and illusions that beset you when you try to walk the mystical path. You may experience this as your dream reality where, on the astral plane, you explore possible actions that can fulfill your destiny and face what blocks them. This is the world of synchronicity, of intuition and illusion, of deeply submerged fears, and even instinctual terror—where you learn to function in the realm of the subconscious. Through the imagination, you can objectify your subjective experience, or it can become mere delusion.

When you embody the Moon, others see you as walking in the dreamtime, for you are attuned to the unconscious currents that flow from past lives evolving into future ones. You function as an oracular sybil in whom madness is suspect. You assist others to cross over into the land of the dead. You must learn, like shellfish, to digest the debris from your past, cleansing the waters of unconscious habits, so as to emerge on the path, walk bravely between the needs of instinct and domestication that "dog" you, past the gates of intellect and technology, to the heights of spiritual intuition. The Moon signifies the mystery and magic of the astral world, where reality is first imagined and genes mutate to evolve new forms.

Sandalwood (*Santalum album*)—(Water, Venus, Jupiter, and Neptune, Pisces)
Sandalwood is a complex spiritual oil that can have many different associations—in tarot, from the Empress to the Sun—yet it has certain qualities that make its placement with the Moon unquestionable. The scent (called *chandana* in Hindi) is said to induce the calm sought by all the spiritualities of India. The oil appears only in trees that are over twenty-five years old. As a "hemiparasite," it uses octopus-like suckers to draw its nutrients from the

roots of neighboring trees and plants. Thus it bleeds its host like a vampire, eventually causing the host's death. A traditional Tantric perfume, its smell is like that of the human pheromone, alpha androsterole.

Sandalwood is filled with paradox. It frees you from material attachments through its qualities of imperishability and lasting value. For serious meditation and spiritual practices, it quiets sexual energies and creates a sacred space and mood for religious ritual, yet it is also known as an aphrodisiac. It can help cure frigidity and impotence when the problem is more psychological than physical by creating a sense of deep relaxation and a loosening of mental boundaries. It enhances creative activity by producing feelings of happiness and joy and stimulating the imagination, yet it sedates and generates feelings of quiet contentment by spreading an aura of peace. It is grounding, quieting to the conscious mind, and excellent for past-life regression.

Marjoram (*Origanum majorana, Marjorana hortensis*)— (Water/Air, Venus, Pisces/Libra)

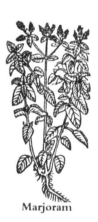

Marjoram

A favorite herb of the ancient Greeks, called "joy of the mountain," it was planted on graves so the ancestors would sleep in peace. It is sacred to Venus, for it takes away the fear of love, yet it is known as a sexual nerve sedative. Comforting and warming, it eases loneliness and grief, and since it deadens the emotions, is helpful when a partner has died. It is also helpful in periods of celibacy. The Prophet Muhammad recommended it for anyone who had lost the sense of smell, but it also sedates the senses, raising the sensory thresholds so that you can digest and process what you have already taken in. It alleviates tension, allays anxieties, and quiets mental chatter, causing drowsiness—and is therefore good for insomnia. It relieves high blood pressure, rheumatism, arthritis, and menstrual cramps, having a subtle valium-like effect. In astral work, it reduces fear and being distracted by delusional effects or feeling trapped by your emotions, while helping you to absorb the meaning of your experiences.

Essence of Tarot

Scott Cunningham says it unifies the psychic and conscious aspects of mind necessary for success in rituals where you enter an altered state.

Melissa (or Lemon Balm) (*Melissa officinalis*) [!]—(Water, Jupiter and Neptune, Pisces)

Melissa chases away dark thoughts and melancholy. Paracelsus called it the "Elixir of Life," and in southern Europe it is known as "heart's delight." Generally soothing and relaxing to a raging mind and emotions, it is good for insomnia, nightmares, shock and grief, and comforts the bereaved. It helps you accept divine will, bringing acceptance and understanding when someone you love is dying. With its help, you can face perils with calm sensitivity. It regulates both ovulatory cycles and thyroid activity. Bees love it (hence the name, which means "bee"), keeping them content in their hives and likewise helping groups draw together for work and meditation. It helps you to remember past lives. It strengthens the nerves, brain, and memory, as well as heart, womb, and digestive system. Its uplifting sense of joy is followed by a quiet peace.

Just a hint of ***Lemon*** (*Citrus limonum*) or ***Lemon Verbena*** (*Lippia citriodora*) may be substituted or exotic flowers like ***Honeysuckle*** (*Lonicera caprifolium*)—(Water, Jupiter)—for weight loss, prosperity, developing and aiding intuition, psychic perception, and yearning and empathy; ***Gardenia*** (*Gardenia* spp.)—(Water, Moon, Pisces)—for peace, love, and spirituality; or ***Violet*** (*Viola odorata*)—(Water, Jupiter)—for beauty and the transitory qualities of life. Violet also aids sleep and heightens spirituality and gives protection for hypersensitivity and for those who are shy.

19—The Sun (Fire, Sun)

The Sun is about affirming life and your own unique personhood. It is a reconciliation of all parts of the self—resulting in a joyous, radiant sense of well-being. When you believe in yourself, acknowledge your achievements, and focus on your goals, you find that success follows close behind. Wherever the Sun shines, hidden facts and motivations are revealed, and everything is laid bare, out in the open. When you embody Sun energy, others see you as a creative leader filled with youthful optimism and enthusiasm. You dazzle and shine and share your happiness with others. Yet, as with the physical sun, you can get "burned out" and exhausted, or you can scorch others with your unrelenting ego and self-assurance. Others may look for a spot of shade to shelter their sensitivities and secrets from your piercing rays that see into everything. The Sun represents the archetype of the child and of rebirth. It celebrates all new beginnings. The bright aroma of the Sun essence is like a winter holiday morning.

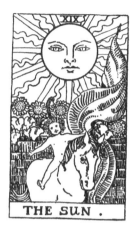

Cinnamon Leaf (not Bark) (*Cinnamomum zeylanicum*)[!]—(Fire, Sun)
The Arabian priests who gathered cinnamon created a myth to keep others from doing so in which they claimed that it could only be obtained from the nests of the phoenix in the land of Bacchus in marshes guarded by winged serpents and bats who attacked one's eyes. The season's first bundles were dedicated to the sun. Like the phoenix who rises from its own ashes, cinnamon represents rebirth. Creating an atmosphere of warmth and welcome, it has been a traditional scent of the winter solstice, welcoming back the sun/son. It promotes blood circulation and increases temperature, so strengthens the heart and nervous system, stimulating physical energy and psychic awareness. Used in Egypt for embalming, it was thought to arouse the physical senses. It promotes joy, prosperity, money and success in business, and creativity. It is a charismatic aroma, drawing others into your energy field, so has been used as an aphrodisiac. It helps bring memories (especially from childhood) into the light of consciousness. *Cassia* (*Cinnamomum cassia*) may be substituted.

Mandarin (*or Tangerine*) (*Citrus reticulata* or *C. nobilis*)—(Fire, Sun, Leo)
This favorite gift of the Chinese mandarins (from whence its name) is a solar oil similar to orange, but it adds an air of youth and freshness and has

been called the "little sun of the heart." Children love its gentle and mild yet refreshing scent. According to Monika Jünneman, it brings brightness into life and lightens small tasks, minor affairs, and lesser matters. Its air of happiness subtly inspires and strengthens you, and its ability to relax you can help with sudden shocks. It is especially good for experiencing the child within you and for whenever you need to look at the bright side of things. It also helps you to absorb things more easily and to expel negative emotions. It is freeing and opening. Use especially for easing maidens through menarche and during pregnancy.

Frankincense (aka Olibanum) (*Boswellia carterii*)[!]—(Fire, Sun, Aries/Leo)
Highly valued in Egypt beginning over 5,000 years ago, it was produced by the Sabians in Punt as a hereditary craft. It was the major incense of the ancient Middle East, used for rituals and funerals where its golden color equated it with the sun, and it equaled or exceeded the value of precious metals and gems. It was also used medicinally to treat a wide range of ailments. Well known as the gift of the Magi at the birth of Jesus, it heightens awareness of spiritual realms, promotes a meditative state, and is unparalleled for opening to cosmic energies, thus deepening your religious experience. When burned, it expands the subconscious and awakens ecstatic energy sources. Its elevating, warming, and soothing effect drives away obsessions, fears, and anxieties, reducing stress and tension. It seems to release you from the cares of the material world, allows you to let go of past transgressions, and alleviates guilt with a sense of divine forgiveness. You gain a sense of personal space that allows for attunement with your highest spiritual aspirations.

20—Judgement (Water, Pluto)

Judgement is about awakening your ability to transcend limitations. It is an epiphany or recognition that creates total change. It reflects on the struggle of each generation of humanity for consciousness and identity, for a voice

The Tarot Oils

of its own. It signifies what "calls" you, whether a vocation, intellectual idea, or great truth—and may require a "crossroads" decision. Judgement hearkens you to the real meaning of your existence, so you can no longer deny your fate. But Judgement is also about using personal judgement to impose control, about calling the tune and making others dance to it. Judgement is criticism, both given and received. It awakens you to your own conscience, asking forgiveness and the chance to atone for your sins. When you embody Judgement, you powerfully affect others through the force of your personality and your values, or you give yourself over, unconditionally, to a greater will. You may also become a spokesperson for the needs of the masses. These contrary meanings of Judgement all point to the liberating call of spirit. The diffused aroma of Judgement essence is reminiscent of fine pipe tobacco.

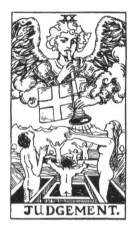

Basil (*Ocimum basilicum*)[!]—(Fire, Mars and Pluto, Scorpio)
The name of this plant means "royal" or "kingly," indicating its association with power and authority. In India, being sacred, it was tended as a household windowsill plant in the name of deceased family members. Associated with opposing qualities, basil epitomizes paradox: love and hate, sacred and evil, antidote and poison. On one hand, it is good for "the stryking of a sea dragon," and on the other, it was thought to breed scorpions in the brain. Yet it opens the gates of heaven to the pious, as depicted on the tarot card. A 16th-century saying was, "The smell of Basil taketh away sorrowfulness and maketh a man

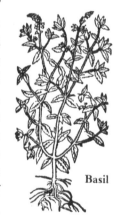

merry and glad." This goes along with its stimulating effect that sharpens senses and concentration while clarifying the intellect and strengthening the nerves. Thus it is good for decision-making. In magic, it is said to attract money.

Pennyroyal (*Mentha pulegium or Hedeoma pulegioides*)[!!]—(Fire/Water, Mars and Pluto, Scorpio)
The name means "royal fleabane" or "poison for the king's fleas." It is an excellent bug repellent and relieves the pain of bites and stings. It also promotes menstruation and is an abortifacient—but beware, it can also hurt or kill the mother (the oil used internally is toxic!). Witches made it into a brew that caused double vision, perhaps to see both sides of an issue. The aroma helps to prevent seasickness during travel and it stills dizziness. It clears the conscious mind and eases mental confusion when trying to make a decision. Since it repels negative thought-forms, Navajo medicine men chewed its seeds and then blew their breath into the patient's face or afflicted part to drive out evil. Gurudas recommends it for resting after hard labor and for anchoring the soul's forces in the physical body.

Anise or Aniseed (*Pimpinella anisum*)[!!]—(Air, Mercury and Pluto)
Anise relieves stress from overwork and overcomes emotional heartache. It is an aphrodisiac in that it stimulates the sex glands. It brings up hidden fears and helps to release guilt and ease the sting of criticism, so that you don't stress yourself into such emotionally based ailments as headaches, indigestion, asthma, colic, impotence/frigidity, or painful periods. Anise liquor is used during voodoo rituals to anoint the heads of initiates to open them to spirit, and an anointing oil is used for foretelling the future because it induces clairvoyance and energizes the brain. In smoking mixtures, it works as an

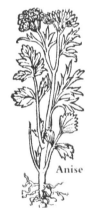
Anise

expectorant, again bringing up stuff that we've breathed in. Anise also attracts fish—perhaps as an aid to fertility.

21—The World (Earth/Air, Saturn)

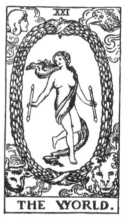

The World card is about the dance of nature, of which William Blake spoke: "Every Tree/And Flower & Herb soon fill the air with an innumerable Dance/Yet all in order sweet & lovely." Saturn promises you that you can have all the bounty of the physical world, that you are, in fact, at its center, with its gifts at your disposal. Your task is to recognize your freedom within this bounty so that you are not bound by it but can bring its beauty and wealth with you when you travel through the cosmos. This image describes how you locate yourself in time and space (the four seasons and directions—as indicated by the eagle, angel, bull, and lion), applying the elements with grace and precision. When you embody the World, others see you as dancing on your limitations, accepting boundaries, but also creating more than meets the eye. On the problematic side, you may be feeling restricted or that your energies are being uncomfortably contained. Overall, you integrate male and female characteristics in your personal expression and present a truly wholistic perspective. The World represents the concept of giving birth to yourself.

Vetiver (*Vetiveria zizanoides*)—(Earth, Saturn and Venus, Capricorn)
This oil comes from roots that spread like brambles deep within the earth. Woven into fans and sprayed with water, they provide a cooling and refreshing breeze in hot, humid countries. Vetiver is a fixative and thus is earthy, practical, and sustaining. It helps you to set both psychic and physical boundaries, protect your home, resist temptations, and gives you a sense

of rootedness. It affirms your connection with Mother Earth and her life-giving energy, which you use to get what you want out of life. A source of vital energy and regeneration, it is warm and stimulating, tending to relax deeply held tensions and fears. It protects those who are oversensitive by creating a psychic shield. It is good for menopause and aging skin and fortifies in you a sense of dignity and wholeness.

Oakmoss (*Evernia prunastri*)—(Earth, Venus and Saturn, Taurus/Capricorn). This definitely energizes you for working with nature spirits. It creates a sense of security, while enhancing your sense of personal prosperity. Medicinally it has been used to treat respiratory complaints and sinus congestion. It puts a cap on runaway emotions, loose talk, and secrets. In money magic, it increases cash flow toward you while keeping other assets from flowing away from you. When exploring spiritual or astral states, use it for securely grounding yourself.

The Minor Arcana Essence Oils

There are several ways to determine essential oils for the Minor Arcana:

1. Select a Minor Arcana card for which you want an oil. Go to the Elements group in the chart called "Astrological Correspondences: Elements, Planets, and Signs" on page 60. Pick one or more oils from the Elements group that correspond to the card's suit. (For Wands, use any oil[s] from the Fire group; for Cups, use Water; for Swords, use Air; and for Pentacles, use Earth.) Look up the oil descriptions in "The 22 Major Arcana Tarot Oils" section, which begins on page 64, until you find one whose characteristics go best with the meaning of the card. For instance, for the 7 of Cups, you would look at the oils in the Elements group next to Water. Upon looking up the characteristics of mugwort, you might pick it for its qualities of bringing dreams and visions.

The Tarot Oils

2. You can use the root number of a card and then relate it to its corresponding Major Arcana card and tarot oil.

MAJOR ARCANA SUBSTITUTIONS FOR MINOR ARCANA CARDS	
Minor Arcana Root Number	**Major Arcana Substitutions**
Aces	1-Magician, 19-Sun
2's	2-High Priestess, 11-Justice (or Strength), 20-Judgement
3's	3-Empress, 12-Hanged One, 21-World
4's	4-Emperor, 13-Death
5's	5-Hierophant, 14-Temperance
6's	6-Lovers, 15-Devil
7's	7-Chariot, 16-Tower
8's	8-Strength (or Justice), 17-Star
9's	9-Hermit, 18-Moon
10's	10-Wheel of Fortune, 19-Sun
Kings	4-Emperor
Queens	3-Empress
Knights/Princes	7-Chariot
Pages/Princesses	8-Strength

3. Make your own associations between the Major Arcana and Minor Arcana. For instance, I associate the 2 of Cups with The Lovers (based on the quality of loving affinity common to both), or the 6 of Wands with The Chariot (based on their mutual aura of victory), or the 8 of Cups with The Moon (based on the idea of the "night journey" in both), or the 10 of Swords with Death (with the idea of release and transformation). Try your own associations in this same manner.

112

Essence of Tarot

4. Use the following chart of suggested correspondences:

THE 56 MINOR ARCANA ESSENCE OILS		
Fire	**Ace of Wands**	Cinnamon
Water	**Ace of Cups**	Roman Chamomile
Air	**Ace of Swords**	Lemongrass
Earth	**Ace of Pentacles**	Vetivert
Mars in *Aries*	**2 of Wands**	Ginger
Venus in *Cancer*	**2 of Cups**	Rose Geranium
Moon in *Libra*	**2 of Swords**	Palmarosa
Jupiter in *Capricorn*	**2 of Pentacles**	Nutmeg
Sun in *Aries*	**3 of Wands**	Frankincense
Mercury in *Cancer*	**3 of Cups**	Lemon
Saturn in *Libra*	**3 of Swords**	Myrrh
Mars in *Capricorn*	**3 of Pentacles**	Juniper Berry
Venus in *Aries*	**4 of Wands**	Myrtle
Moon in *Cancer*	**4 of Cups**	Camphor
Jupiter in *Libra*	**4 of Swords**	Bergamot
Sun in *Capricorn*	**4 of Pentacles**	Patchouli
Saturn in *Leo*	**5 of Wands**	Pine
Mars in *Scorpio*	**5 of Cups**	Marjoram
Venus in *Aquarius*	**5 of Swords**	Peppermint
Mercury in *Taurus*	**5 of Pentacles**	Thyme
Jupiter in *Leo*	**6 of Wands**	Laurel
Sun in *Scorpio*	**6 of Cups**	Mandarin
Mercury in *Aquarius*	**6 of Swords**	Cypress
Moon in *Taurus*	**6 of Pentacles**	Cardamom

The Tarot Oils

THE 56 MINOR ARCANA ESSENCE OILS (continued)

Mars in *Leo*	**7 of Wands**	Pennyroyal
Venus in *Scorpio*	**7 of Cups**	Mugwort
Moon in *Aquarius*	**7 of Swords**	Eucalyptus
Saturn in *Taurus*	**7 of Pentacles**	Anise
Mercury in *Sagittarius*	**8 of Wands**	Wintergreen
Saturn in *Pisces*	**8 of Cups**	Spikenard
Jupiter in *Gemini*	**8 of Swords**	Clove
Sun in *Virgo*	**8 of Pentacles**	Petitgrain
Moon in *Sagittarius*	**9 of Wands**	Cedar
Jupiter in *Pisces*	**9 of Cups**	Sandalwood
Mars in *Gemini*	**9 of Swords**	Lavender
Venus in *Virgo*	**9 of Pentacles**	Spearmint
Saturn in *Sagittarius*	**10 of Wands**	Sage
Mars in *Pisces*	**10 of Cups**	Coriander
Sun in *Gemini*	**10 of Swords**	Rue
Mercury in *Virgo*	**10 of Pentacles**	Clary Sage
Aries	**King of Wands**	Black Pepper
Cancer	**King of Cups**	Labdanum
Libra	**King of Swords**	Fir
Capricorn	**King of Pentacles**	Basil
Leo	**Queen of Wands**	Rosemary
Scorpio	**Queen of Cups**	Ylang-ylang
Aquarius	**Queen of Swords**	Niaouli
Taurus	**Queen of Pentacles**	Bois de Rose
Sagittarius	**Prince of Wands**	Hyssop
Pisces	**Prince of Cups**	Carrot
Gemini	**Prince of Swords**	Dill
Virgo	**Prince of Pentacles**	Oakmoss
Root of Fire	**Princess of Wands**	Sassafras
Root of Water	**Princess of Cups**	Vanilla (Balsam Peru)
Root of Air	**Princess of Swords**	Storax (Benzoin)
Root of Earth	**Princess of Pentacles**	Caraway Seed

CHAPTER 6

Magic and Ritual

"Magic is the exploration of the essence and power of all things."
—Psellus, 11th-century Byzantine philosopher

Making Magic

Earlier, when I discussed aroma imaging (patterning or reprogramming using scents), I was really talking about *making magic*. After surveying hundreds of definitions of magic from some of the greatest authorities of the Western magical tradition, I think that Aleister Crowley still sums it up best: "Magick is the science and art of causing change to occur in conformity with will," with its updated corollary: "Magic is the art of changing consciousness at will."[1] This means that with directed will, you can accomplish your intent. But as the Golden Dawn taught, it takes not only will but also imagination.

First you must *imagine* the end result of your purpose or intent. Using imagination, you visualize a picture of what you want in all its details. The tarot cards can greatly help you to clarify that picture, and scent brings it vividly to mind through associated memories. According to Rousseau, "Smell is the sense of the imagination"—not only because it has the property of refreshing the memory but also because it does so with such artistry and scope. Essential oils can link us directly with such moments of imaginative recall.

The other important element is emotion—the feeling that underlies the desire to accomplish your intent. Emotion is the engine that drives the will.

Fear blocks the positive flow of feelings, whether fear of failure or fear of success. Essential oils—as the pheromones of the plants—are, simply, liquid desire. Desire fuels the process, and you can kindle it with an affirmative emotion—also by using essential oils—at its most physiological level. Then it is a matter of directing your single-focused will upon an image clearly and precisely visualized as already accomplished on the etheric plane.

As MacGregor Mathers, a founder of the Golden Dawn, explained: "Magic is the science of the control of the secret forces of nature." And essential oils bring us into immediate contact with those secret forces. They are not just signs pointing to a truth; they participate in the etheric reality that they signify. They are believed to have an ethereal counterpart easily detectable in the world of Spirit. Since the molecules of scent are so close to the intangible, they reach a likewise intangible, psychic, or etheric plane more readily than any other medium.

Oils change the way the mind works, so that it is soon not a matter of "control," as Mathers and medieval magicians believed, but one of alignment and accord. As Florence Farr found, magic "unlimits experience," so that we can name our powers and realize our wisdom.

Ritual is merely the acting out of this process, using physical symbols of the things desired and enclosing us within a sacred space in which the transformation can be safely performed. According to modern ritualist Kay Turner, "In the context of ritual, women are creating a space in which to feel better, to feel more, to feel the past as well as the future. Perhaps most important is the way in which ritual upholds and celebrates the validity of feeling as a mode of revelation, communication, and transvaluation."[2]

You see, ultimately the goal of all real magic is to harmonize with the Divine, or as Crowley put it: "The goal of magick is the knowledge and conversation of the Holy Guardian Angel." It involves transforming your consciousness from an outer state of awareness to an inner state of awareness—redirecting your experience to the part of yourself that is united with Spirit. The association of scent with ethereal and otherworldly realities affords you a glimpse of your most essential nature and (with the "odor of sanctity" and the ability to rise, as do angels) an ability to greet the gods. And it is the Major Arcana of the tarot that provides a map of the way. The goal of true magic is that your will and the will of the Divine be one and the same. The essential oils, as part of the secret forces of nature, can be your guides and teachers.

About Rituals

Now we come to what you *do* with the oils. According to Dion Fortune, any act performed with intention becomes a ritual. Therefore all of the techniques I suggest here become rituals if you perform them with focused intention. Without awareness, we have only empty gestures—so it is up to you to turn mere actions into magic.

The first four cards of the Major Arcana describe the magical process.

The Magician card depicts total attention concentrated on a single purpose, while **The High Priestess** demonstrates how to relax and center the emotions in perfect balance. **The Empress** shows how imagination creates a desire—image filled with sensory detail, and **The Emperor** projects the force of will—balanced by impersonal emotion—into the desire-image you have formed.

You do not have to do anything elaborate to create a ritual; or, on the other hand, you can employ all kinds of magical tools, such as charts of the hours and sacred circles of salt guarded in the four directions by flaming pentacles.[3] Elaborate formal rituals, however, can intensify the effectiveness of your work, because every part of yourself is brought to bear on gathering materials and preparing for the ritual; the formalities keep you focused during the process and ensure that all your personal senses and symbolic triggers are brought into specific alignment with planetary and cosmic forces. Still, I must admit that spontaneous rituals, using the objects at hand, have been among the most powerful experiences I have personally known. In any case, remember that aligning with the forces of nature has more to do with recognizing and feeling them in and around yourself than it does with following rules and traditions.

Magic and Ritual

Ritual is a tool for patterning consciousness to obtain the results you want. Its purpose is personal transformation. As we have already seen, smell is one of the most powerful ways of patterning your consciousness because it directly evokes memories and emotional and physical responses. Through ritual, we transform our experiences into an encounter with the Divine. Ritual is a technique for contacting spiritual forces that can impart their vibrational energy to our work in the material world.

Author and occultist Helena Blavatsky suggested that in ritual the above and the below must be brought together and made to act harmoniously. First, she says, we perceive the essence of things in the light of nature. Then, using the soul powers of that essence, we produce material things from the unseen universe. As previously discussed, essential oils are the soul force of the vegetable kingdom and are the concentrated energy of the sun spirit, manifested in terms of the specific characteristics of the plant. By evoking[4] those energies and purposefully directing them, you can produce material results (including the psycho-spiritual ones) on the physical plane. In some cultures, the effect of plant odors is even more direct. According to anthropologist David Howes, writing on New Guinea magic and olfaction, "for a spell to work [in the Kwoma culture] it must be carried on a smell." In other words, "the power of a spell is in its *smell*, its aroma, not simply its verbal structure."[5] One of the (many) reasons our Western culture is so cut off from our source on this planet is that we have forgotten the power of smell, or we use it in only the most materially based manipulative ways.

The media for the transfer of energy in a ritual are, therefore, myth, symbol, and smell, because through them you evoke the corresponding energies. They link the above and the below, the macrocosm and the microcosm, the Divine and the human, the objective and the subjective. They form a channel between your unconscious and the power behind the form, so that you can make contact with it. They are energy transformers converting divine essences into ideas, and ideas into images, and images into words or objects. Conversely, material objects can lead you back again to essence. Thus, by manipulating the words or objects, you can reach behind them, eventually back to the essence itself.

Symbols and smells, then, allow energy exchanges among different vibrational levels to take place. Because they extend back to the Divine, all symbols can link you to spiritual truth. For instance, the physical rose represents the beauty of the female genitals (where the stage of bloom indicates the female maturity), which in turn stands for the Goddess—but behind this is the allure of the purely generative force, and behind that—in the image of multiple petals and the center—we have the many in the one. To smell a rose is to link with Divinity.

Myth consists of symbols strung together to tell a story, which also describes a psychological process, so that the physical story is but a reflection of a spiritual one—like that told in tarot. By discovering the myths of plants and odors, you can reconnect with the ancient knowledge (secret only because forgotten) of the power of aroma. Ritual is the reenactment of myth, remembered through scent.

So, within the ritual setting, you name and invoke the powers you desire. These powers exist both within you and without. Then, via symbols, you transfer the power from the unconscious or archetypal realm to the conscious, physical realm. Knowledge of the correspondences between object, myth, symbol, and meaning allow you to generate calculable results. The more you know about their hidden relationships, the more you can draw from those sources of power with your intent.

Tarot cards stand for a multitudinous range of myths, archetypes, and psychological states. As author Kathleen Raine points out: "The Tarot symbols . . . [give] the freedom to evoke, in their living essence, those personifying spirits which by different nations have been variously named."[6] Thus the High Priestess can represent Isis, Astarte, moon-crowned Hathor, the oracular sybils, a female pope, the wise woman within, or the tarot reader or querent. Tarot cards are incredibly flexible, so that one time we perceive one association, say, of the Hierophant as wise and generous, and another time we see him differently, as rigid and dogmatic.

The magical and transformative energies within essential oils can be discovered through three main sources: the myths told about them; a physical resemblance of the plant to another thing, which results in a related meaning

Magic and Ritual

being assigned to both (known as the doctrine of signatures); and through the ways in which they work physiologically on the mind and body—which may or may not also be indicated by the other two. Thus an essential oil that is resistant to pests can be used to keep psychic or human pests away. An oil that is good for states of panic is related to Pan from which the word originally came, and therefore we might look at the myths of Pan for a way to transform panic into mirth (see The Devil card).

Outline for Ritual

Personally, I rarely work from tightly scripted rituals, and therefore I am not going to give you any specifically detailed rituals. However, I do use a kind of outline, and I will share with you the basic form I have developed. I prefer "suggested" frameworks and techniques within which transformation can take place, changing not only the participants but the ritual itself. In the next chapter, I will suggest some things you might choose to do to ritualize your experience with tarot and essential oils.

Here is the outline I use for creating ritual. You can also use "The Creative Work-Cycle Spread" in chapter 8 to help you design your ritual. The first two steps are preparatory and consist of questions to answer before you begin.

1. What is the ritual for? What do you want to empower or align with, and what do you want to transform, create, or draw to you? This is your purpose or intent. It should be clearly stated.

2. What do you need to do to prepare for this ritual? Consider the time, astrological aspects, season, place, who you want to be there (both physically and on the astral planes).

   An altar is where we go to alter our consciousness. It exists wherever we focus our consciousness and need not be physical. What materials, tools, or symbols do you want on your altar?

120   *Essence of Tarot*

Is there a myth or story that parallels your intent? Do you want to reenact some archetypal human experience?

3. Gather together everything you will need.

4. Purify yourself and the space. Traditionally, this may involve a cleansing bath and/or smudging with incense (cedar or sage burned in a shell is excellent), sprinkling with salt water, or shaking a rattle to release and clear stuck energies.

5. Create a sacred circle. Often this is done by calling on the four directions, casting a circle, and doing an initial grounding and centering exercise. It can be done simply by directing your breath through your imagination to extend and solidify your aura, creating a kind of bubble around you or a group. Focus your energy within the circle using chants, drums, grounding visualizations, etc.

6. Invoke the presence of whatever energy whose power you wish to draw on. This may be a goddess, god, creator, mythological figure, or personal guides and helpers. State your purpose. Charge any implements you may want to use, and bless objects on the altar. Sometimes telling the story of why each object is present is a good way to center on your purpose. (e.g., "I have chosen to use oil of nutmeg for this ritual in order to banish mental fatigue and lethargy, and to bring me prosperity and optimistic thoughts. It always reminds me of . . .")

7. The work:

   a. Before you can create, you often have to *banish*; therefore, many rituals will include at this point a banishing or releasing of whatever is keeping you from the changes you desire. This may include getting rid of unwanted energy, emotions, behaviors, and memories. This process can be spoken, acted, sung, danced, or written out on paper and burned. (An example of a banishing myth is the story of the goddess—Persephone or Inanna—entering the underworld as the Hermit and being stripped of everything she carries, leaving behind her light, her staff, her cloak.) You may need to cry, grieve, or acknowledge old wounds. This should be followed by a healing and balancing of the chakras or energy field.

b. Energy abhors a vacuum. Now you have an open space in which to create what you want to bring in to your life or to transform. To make your images clear and precise, use stories (i.e., the Goddess reemerging from the underworld can be envisioned as the Star) and visualizations—along with chants, songs, enactments, or the making of charms and talismans. Involve all your senses, if possible, by touching, tasting, smelling, hearing, and seeing things that symbolically correspond to your desire.

8. Empower or charge your work. Using visualization, breath, light, and sound (vibrating the syllable "OM," for instance), imagine a cone of energy building over your work and connecting with the powers you have invoked. It swirls around, perhaps like an upside-down whirlpool, until you release it to spin off into the cosmos.

9. Immediately ground the energy, bringing the charge to earth and thus into manifestation—usually by using your arms, hands, and perhaps a wand to move energy from the "working" down to touch the earth. Imagine the energy moving through you like a conduit and taking root in the ground.

10. Follow with a period of silent gratitude and thanksgiving, opening yourself to receive any messages from the "ground" of your being. Perhaps there is something that is not yet finished or another chant to be sung, acknowledgement made, or a step to be completed.

11. Thank and dismiss those energies whose presence you have invoked.

12. Release the guardians of the four directions and open the circle.

13. Review the ritual soon afterward and again later, after a period of time. Discern what worked and what didn't. Evaluate what you learned. Note things you will do differently next time.

Once you understand the steps, they can be quite simple and almost automatic, leaving your attention clearly focused on your intention and upon the movement of the energy and the presences you have invoked.

Follow these simplified steps for an informal, spontaneous ritual:

1. Take several deep breaths with which you center yourself, create sacred space, and invoke your spirit helpers.

2. Do your work, charge it, release it, ground, and receive.

3. Thank and release the energies present and, with a specific and definite act, reenter "normal" space.

Besides these steps, there are two things that especially express the essence of a ritual: offering and sacrifice.

An offering consists of something you donate as thanksgiving for the opportunities within the ritual—to learn, change, grow, and experience harmony with the forces of nature and the Divine. It is an acknowledgement of the continuity and connection of life and often involves a "return" of something to the symbolical place from which it came. For instance, when you take from a living plant for magical purposes, you should not only ask permission but you should also leave something behind. Traditionally this may be a bit of cornmeal or tobacco or a small crystal. When you drink from a cup, a drop should be offered first to Mother Earth. In a group ritual, the offering may be food brought for everyone to share (remember to set a plate for those you have invoked from the astral planes).

Some offerings are sacrifices. Sacrifice means that in order to create a change you must be willing to give up something. This can be as simple as giving up the sympathy of others in order to be healed or giving up sleeping late in order to have the time for quiet meditation. In a sense, by letting something go, you create space in your life for something new to come in. Sacrifices that involve physical pain and wanton destruction are completely unnecessary. In finding a symbol for your sacrifice, think of recycling, for what you sacrifice may be another's gift.

Magic and Ritual

For instance, in a rite of passage, you can let go of something that marks you as the person you previously were. A young girl going through menarche could give a stuffed animal or a favorite outfit to a younger child. You may also sacrifice your personal time and energy to do something for others. Remember that the transformative aspect of symbol means you can make sacrifices symbolically, as Pythagoras did when he instituted the burning of incense instead of animals.

Be conscious of the everyday sacrifices upon which your welfare depends: the sacrifice of plants for food and medicine, trees for houses and paper, creatures for their flesh and byproducts. These are the things we give up in order to live our lives as we do. But sometimes you should examine what you sacrifice in the rituals of life, in order to determine whether you could beneficially transform some of your daily rituals through the use of symbol instead of substance.

Although you may carefully plan a ritual beforehand, leave room for unpredictable transformations that may change your ritual in some way. For instance, in a workshop, we once did a ritual to keep it from raining the next day. Yet during the ritual (in which we laid out tarot cards from many different decks to describe what we wanted), our intent changed—we felt that the weather was doing exactly what it should do, and we came, within the ritual itself, to respect its wisdom. The next day, it rained whenever we needed to be indoors, and the sun shone warm and welcoming whenever we needed to be outdoors. Anyone involved in a ritual may receive messages and feel forces that want to move through them. Being transformed, they will want and need a way to express these forces, so some rituals should allow for such personal experiences and build on them. There is a place for formal ceremonial rituals that have evolved over decades and centuries and millennia, but we cannot explore these here with the attention they demand.

Before we move on to the techniques and rituals for working with the tarot and essential oils, I will mention several forms in which you may use the oils and how to prepare your own set of anointing oils.

The Magical Forms of Essential Oils

The magical use of scent takes several forms: 1) incenses, 2) environmental diffusion, 3) oils or unguents used for anointing and bathing, 4) teas, and 5) herbal amulets. I won't discuss the last two forms here except to say that regarding herbal teas (*tisanes*), their psychological and healing properties sometimes have as much to do with the oil molecules rising with the steam as in the drink itself; and regarding amulets, you can add essential oils to herb mixtures before wrapping them in cloth, just as you add oils to enliven potpourris.

Incense

Perfume literally means "through the smoke." The burning of incense, called thurification, has always been part of magical and spiritual ceremonies around the world. At first the incense merely covered the smell of sacrificed flesh, but later, with Pythagoras as a primary advocate, the sacrifice of plants replaced that of animals, and the gods were pleased. Burning was an act of transmutation in which plant material changed into ash and ethereal odor; in other words, separated into its physical and spiritual components. It is the release of essential oil molecules into the air by heat that creates the scents for which incense is known. Nevertheless, incense creates ethereal roads (visually seen in the smoke) upon which a supplicant travels to meet the gods and via which the gods can send down their gifts. (Similarly, tarot oils may be blended with corresponding herbs and then burned on incense coals to create pathways to the tarot archetypes.)

Incense serves the ceremonial purpose of cleansing or purifying objects, the environment, and ourselves of inappropriate energies and then attuning all these to the vibration of the spiritual agency being invited. It results in the feeling of sacredness—of being set apart from the mundane world—so essential to inner work. It elevates our spirits and helps us focus inwardly and meditatively. Prayers may be sent to heaven on the smoke rising from incense or a ceremonial pipe, but it is the sweetness of the scent that makes our prayers and supplications acceptable to Spirit.

Magic and Ritual

During periods of plague and other epidemics, the disinfectant and antibiotic qualities of essential oils, released during the burning of incense in religious ceremonies, removed germs from the air—actually helping those who attended church to heal and be protected from disease, which in ancient times was seen as effectively exorcising demons and jinn.

Water Sprays / Aroma Lamps / Diffusers

These devices can be used to scent your entire environment to correspond with the energy of a tarot card without offending people who are allergic or sensitive to smoke. Also, many scents are impaired by heat, so you obtain more of the vital energy of the oil using these methods. Use essential oils that have not been mixed with a carrier oil.

WATER SPRAYS

One way to release the scent is to mix the essential oils with water and then spray in a fine mist. To make a spray: first fill a six-ounce spray bottle with distilled water. Add 2 to 4 drops of essential oil. Always shake before using, as the oil and water separate. Spray your hair and face for the moisturizing, energizing, and revitalizing effects. This is wonderful on hot days and while riding in non-air-conditioned cars! Use sprays when traveling to revitalize you and to counteract jet lag. Add a little salt to the water, and spray everyone lightly during pre-ritual purification.

WARMING

The second technique is to warm the oils gently so as to release the scent molecules into the air. You can buy aroma lamps or ceramic rings that fit onto light bulbs. In the winter, I scent my office with a small ceramic bowl set on a heater. Use 2 drops of essential oil in ¼ to ½ cup of distilled water for a small room, or as much as 6 to 10 drops of essential oil for a large open room. Whatever your method, don't let the water boil, because it will release the aroma too quickly, and molecular structure changes with heat and decreases the efficacy of some oils.

DIFFUSION

An electric diffuser that pumps a jet of air through a container into which you have placed the oils is the best, and now relatively inexpensive, way of suffusing a room with molecules of scent that have not been harmed by heat. Oils used in diffusers should never be diluted in carrier oils, which will clog the mechanism. Some diffusers can be noisy, so plug one in for about fifteen to twenty minutes before a ritual or meditation, then unplug it when you begin.

Anointing Oils

Oils or unguents for anointing (diluted in carrier oils), on the other hand, can be seen as representing the astral fluid of the kundalini, or the blood of Spirit. The essential oil chosen represents one's aspiration and is absorbed into your body. In its purest state, it is the chrism of grace, the spark of vital life force bestowed by the Divine within Mother Nature, and it represents the ability to unite the spiritual with the physical through the realm of the psyche. An oil works two ways: first you consecrate it to your use, then it consecrates you. *On a magical level, essential oils are pure light translated into terms of desire.* Thus consecration with an oil elevates you into the highest frequencies of the qualities it represents so that you can work with and from that sacred space. And all consecrated oils concentrate your will into your intention. They heighten your consciousness, call to those spirit help-ers with which they have affinity, evoke corresponding emotions, and create the physiological and physical effects that bring about the desired end.

Oils are generally inimical to water: they are slippery and viscous. Being combustible, they are fuels that provide light and heat when ignited. As lubri-cants, they can "oil the way," making your path more easily traversed. In conse-crating an oil, you are spiritually igniting it so as to fuel your intent. The ability of oil to float on water becomes your ability, when consecrated with an oil, to float on or separate yourself temporarily from mundane concerns.

Much of the next three sections describes the preparation of oils for anointing.

Magic and Ritual

Massage Oils

Make yourself some tarot massage oil; use it on your whole body or just a portion. For example, massages can be effectively included in rites of passage and healing rituals. Doing a ritual foot massage for yourself with tarot oils can be a powerful way of opening all your psychic centers and preparing you to walk in the footsteps of the particular tarot archetype you chose. For a two-ounce bottle (enough for three or four full-body massages), use about 15 to 25 drops of essential oil in the carrier oil of your choice or dilute your anointing oil with up to twice as much carrier oil.

Bath Oils

Ritual baths can be for any intention. Some people meditate best in the bath. Traditionally a bath is for psychic cleansing, often as preparation for a specific task.

Mix about a quarter-ounce of a previously made tarot oil of your choice (or 6 to 8 drops of undiluted essential oil) with sea salt, dairy cream, or a small amount of honey. Add this to the hot water in the tub *after* you have filled it so that the healing molecules don't evaporate too quickly. As the steam rises, visualize the departure of any and all impurities that are not in harmony with your intention. Imagine that your intended purpose is soaking deep into your body through your skin and breathe your intention in with the scent.

Colognes and Perfumes

Instead of putting the essential oils in a base of oil, you can create a perfume by using alcohol, but be warned that most people find that for magical work, the alcohol tends to destroy the life force found in natural oils. You can use denatured alcohol or try using alcohol made from grapes. Of course, a true alchemist would distill, in seven stages, their own 200-proof alcohol.[7] For perfume, begin with a base that is about ¾ brandy or cognac and ¼ distilled water. Then add your essential oils to an amount that is about 5 to 10 percent of the total. (If

128   *Essence of Tarot*

you want to eliminate the slight brandy or cognac scent, first pour the alcohol through a coffee filter filled with activated charcoal, as used for filtering water.)

Perfumes are designed with a mixture of oils that give them what is known as a head or top note, a middle or heart note, and a base note, according to a system resembling musical chords. For our purposes, this is not necessary, but for a longer-lasting perfume with multiple layers, any good book on perfumes will tell you how this is done. As with the oil base, you will find these perfumes to be quite different from the commercial variety, which use mostly synthetics.

For magical purposes, a perfume works best when used in social situations. You can use it as plants do—to lure the means of sexual fertilization. You can leave your unique personal mark imprinted on someone's memory and emotions. You can exude self-confidence and boost your own self-esteem. Or you can use a perfume as a magical shield of protection.

When wanting to imprint your scent on another person, don't wear a perfume that they claim to like without first finding out why. If it was because the person's mother or a previous lover wore it, you will only be evoking memories of the other person. Also be sure to connect your scent with the most pleasant of experiences.[8]

When mixing essential oils in a perfume, you will find that the molecules combine over a period of about two to three weeks, yielding a new scent that is their combination. Some scents (the top notes) will evaporate faster, eventually leaving you with the more lasting odors (those known as the fixatives) predominating. Mix your perfumes in small amounts (¼ to ½ oz.) to try them first. Keep careful records of all your experiments and measure carefully so you can reproduce that perfect combination again.

Since anointing oils are one of the most efficient ways of using the tarot cards and the corresponding essential oils, the next chapter will detail exactly how to make your own, either for an individual tarot card or for an entire set of twenty-two oils.

Magic and Ritual

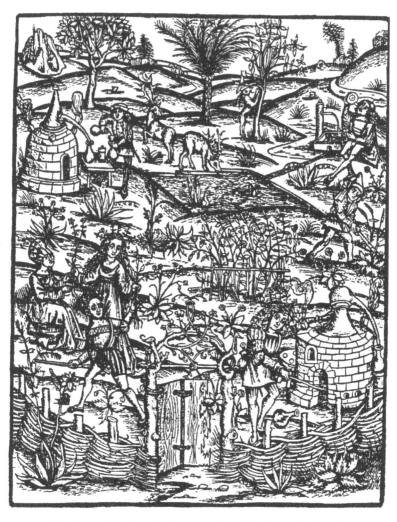

Distillers working in an herb garden. From *Liber de Arte Distillandi*, by Hieronymus Brunschwigk, 1500.

CHAPTER 7

Tarot Oil Techniques

*"Virtue is like precious odours—
most fragrant when they are incensed, or crushed."*
—Francis Bacon, *Of Adversity*

Let us say that you have purchased the essential oils that go with your personality or soul card (see appendix A). Before you combine the oils together to make a tarot oil, you might want to get in contact with the individual oils and their elemental or "angelic" energies to, so to speak, enter the field of their reality. As Monika Jünnemann explains: "Communication with plants is an exchange in the consciousness of love, a balance of give and take which affects all dimensions of being. Plants are one of the forms of life which manifest cosmic consciousness on this earth and every plant we communicate with transmits this cosmic information to us."[1]

Before you begin, review this grounding and centering process that I recommend doing with all the rituals and processes in this book. Whenever I say "ground yourself," this will help you establish an energy connection with the earth and sky.

Grounding and Centering Process

(You may wish to tape these instructions.)

Generally, you will want to sit in a chair, your feet flat on the floor, with your eyes closed. If you sit cross-legged, then you will send energy into the earth through the base of your spinal cord rather than your feet. Take three slow deep breaths, and with each breath feel yourself becoming quieter and more centered within yourself. As you exhale, release the thoughts and cares of the day. For the time being, let go of any concerns you may have. As you inhale, feel your attention riding on your breath into the center of your being. Following your breath as it moves through your body, notice any places where tension exists and release and gently let this tension go.

Then exhale through the soles of your feet into the earth, as if you had roots. When you inhale, allow the rich nourishment and life-giving properties of the earth to rise up through these roots and spread through your body, your veins, and your cells, so that you feel refreshed and revitalized. With each exhalation, feel your roots stretch deeper into the earth, past the topsoil, past the gravel, through the levels of clay, to rock and along the fissures of the rock, reaching deeper, past the underground waterways and the volcanic fires to the very center of the earth. With each inhalation, bring up the deep strength and power of the earth, inhale an awareness of the ages and eternities it took for its formation.

When your roots have curled around a rock at the inmost center of the planet, then bring that feeling of deep-rootedness up as you inhale, filling the center of your being with that security. With your next exhalation, send your breath up through your trunk, stretching out along branches and out the leaves, releasing the dark vitality of the earth to the cosmos. Inhale the light of the sun and bring it down through you, so that on your next exhalation, you send that light energy out through your roots and give it to the earth. Inhale the energies of Mother Earth, bringing them through you again and exhaling them out through your branches, giving them to the cosmos, and from sky above draw the power of light into the earth.

Essence of Tarot

Then simultaneously draw the energies from above and below into your heart, and as you exhale open your heart and give away your breath for the good of all beings. With each breath expand the dimensions of your "give away" until you feel in harmony and connected to everything around you. Bring your intention from your mind into your heart. Make any changes or adjustments necessary to this intention until your heart totally accepts it. If appropriate, you can release your intention into the world on your next breath or keep it in readiness for a later moment of release.

Know that at any time you need to ground your energy again during your work, you can take one to three deep breaths and feel completely centered and secure in your connectedness. At the end of a process, you might want to put your hands, palm down, directly on the ground and let any excess energy drain from you as you re-root yourself.

Communicating with a Plant

If possible, go to a place where the plant is actually growing. If your card is Strength, for instance, then you will want to find rosemary, juniper, or an orange tree. Ground and center yourself. Your eyes may be kept open or closed.

Tell the plants in general what it is that you are doing and what you want from them—for instance, communication, attunement, or knowledge of how to use this plant's essential oil. Call to the plant and wait in silence until you feel some kind of response. Trust your senses, no matter how subtle. If nothing happens, then playfully imagine what would occur if something were to happen. If a specific plant were to draw you, which one would it be? Follow that lead wherever it takes you—as if it were real.

Sit down next to that plant. Imagine you and the plant within a sacred circle, which you can mark out with your finger or a stick or simply in your mind. Within this space, reach out and feel for the aura of the plant itself. Make sure that you are welcome and in accord, then ask if you may take a bit of the plant.

Tarot Oil Techniques

You can assume it is all right if you feel no sense of rejection or "wrongness." Take a flower or leaf and crush it between your fingers to obtain the scent. Ask for the elemental or the angel of the plant to come forward. Its presence will be felt by a subtle change in the space around you. Imagine what it would look like if you could see it, and write down, now or later, all of your perceptions. Now ask the elemental or angel what use you can make of the oil—what it is for—or, perhaps, how it is different from the plant. Be aware that sometimes specific plants have their own agendas that will be different from the rest of the species. Ask if this is so in the information you are receiving. Write everything down. Thank the elemental or angel of the plant and separate yourself from its energies by seeing both your aura and its own aura as separate and whole. Check your grounding, then open the circle. You are done.[2] It is only polite to leave a small offering of some kind: corn meal, tobacco, a crystal, or a penny is fine.

Communicating with an Essential Oil

If your oil is ylang-ylang or black pepper, you may not have the plant around, but you can use a similar process. This time, you will make an astral journey to the "inner reality" of the oil. Playing meditative or environmental music softly in the background will help create a sacred space for your meditation. Put a single drop of your chosen oil on a cotton ball, tissue, or small square of cotton rag paper (watercolor paper works well). (See also the Sufi technique described at the beginning of the section called "Uses for the Tarot Oils" on page 146.) For the time being, just keep it near at hand. Sit comfortably in a chair with your feet flat on the ground. Close your eyes. Center and ground yourself; take a few moments to completely relax the muscles in every part of your body, beginning with your head, moving down your shoulders, arms, chest, legs, and finally relaxing your feet and toes.

Imagine that you are walking along a path through a field or forest. When you are fully present and can feel the path beneath your feet and the air moving through your hair, pick up your cotton ball or paper, keeping your focus

Essence of Tarot

inward, and place it where you can smell it without any effort. Imagine that as you continue along your path, this scent comes wafting to you on the breeze. Follow the scent, letting it lead you until you come upon the plant itself. It may be in a garden, a field of flowers, or even a flowerpot. It may look like the real plant or completely different—for instance, taking on some fantasy form. Whatever its form, accept it. Tell the plant(s) why you have come. Then follow the previous instructions for communicating with a plant, beginning where you sit down next to the plant. When you end the process, make sure you are back in your body and completely grounded before opening your eyes.

An alternate way of exploring the characteristics of an oil is to ask the tarot cards. While smelling the oil as suggested above, spread your tarot cards in a fan, face down, on a table or held in your hand. Draw one card while asking, "What is the message of your essence?" Act as if the oil were speaking directly to you, using this card as its means of communication. What does it say? If necessary, ask for clarification and draw another card, or ask another question such as, "What do you have to offer me?" or "How can I best use you?" Alternately you can ask questions about how to interpret the myths and stories associated with the plant or its essential oil. Continue asking questions and drawing cards at random from the fanned deck until your dialogue feels completed.

Making and Using Tarot Oils

Always use essential oils *externally* and in a diluted form unless you are thoroughly familiar with their healing uses and physical properties. Some oils can cause severe reactions or even be toxic in large amounts, and some are extracted via solvents that leave a toxic residue in the oil. Pregnant women should avoid such oils altogether and use other essential oils in only the lightest concentrations. Anyone with epilepsy or other seizure disorders should also take extreme care, as epileptic and other seizures can be triggered by scent.

Oils for anointing should be in diluted form, with approximately 3 to 5 percent of essential oil in a base of vegetable oil (such as almond, avocado,

Tarot Oil Techniques

hazelnut, sunflower seed, safflower, olive, or jojoba) and with a few drops of natural mixed-tocopherol vitamin E (or wheat germ oil) to act as a preservative and healing agent.

Choosing a Carrier Oil

Oils for anointing or massage are generally made from a base oil that forms the medium or carrier, which is then combined with essential oils to give the desired fragrance. Choose a carrier oil as carefully as you do your essential oils. All oils have their special qualities, but, in general, oils open the emotional body through touch. They help you to get in touch with your potentials, bring them out, and "oil the way" for magic to work. This is why it is so important to be clear about your intentions, both when anointing and when giving or receiving a massage.

Olive oil is traditionally the gift of Minerva, Roman goddess of wisdom, and has been used for centuries in magical workings. Symbolically it represents the peace of the goddess and fruitfulness. In Spain, an olive crop's health and quality was dependent on a husband's fidelity and a woman being master of the house.

The sunflower is known for following the light and mimicking the glory of the sun. Gurudas, who recommends this oil for sunburn, says it amplifies qualities of spiritual leadership in the personality and awakens a man's maternal instinct.

The almond represents first flowering, divine pardon, and compassion, but it is also known as a fertility symbol called "Womb of the World." It provided the wood for Aaron's rod and traditionally means "hope," because its blooming was a harbinger of spring.

Sesame was seen by the Egyptians as a seed of life and was their favorite oil for anointing. The magical formula "open sesame" in many variant folk tales opened closed places like doors, trees, caves, or mountains to reveal great riches. Use it to open your own closed places and reveal your hidden wealth. According to Theophrastus, sesame oil receives rose perfume better than any other.

Other suitable oils include avocado, grape seed, peach and apricot kernel, or safflower.

136   *Essence of Tarot*

Waxes such as beeswax or jojoba can also be used as your carrier, and, traditionally, highly refined animal fats have been used. If you are making up a number of tarot oils that you plan to use over a period of six months or more, then use jojoba oil (actually a vegetable wax), as it never goes rancid.

To make a quarter-ounce bottle (2 dram or 7.4 milliliters) of a tarot oil for anointing purposes, you would use a maximum of 6 to 8 drops of essential oil; less with the cautionary oils. (Suggestion: start with 1 drop of each essential oil; then you have room to adjust relative intensities if necessary.) If using a single essential oil, 3 to 5 drops may be all you need.

This dilution is perfectly safe to use on your skin, although especially sensitive people with allergies could experience a slight reaction (rash or burning sensation). If you have a reaction, wash with cold water and then apply plain vegetable oil as a salve. If you have hypersensitive skin, dilute with half the number of drops given above (resulting in a 2- to 3-percent solution).

To avoid oxidation, store all oils in a cool place, never leaving them in the sun or in a warm location. Although many people insist on amber-colored bottles, this is not necessary if you keep the bottles in a cool, dark place. Clear bottles allow you to see the different colors of the oils. Essential oils themselves are often preservatives, but the carrier oils can go rancid. In general, citrus essences are the most volatile (lasting about 12 to 18 months), then herbs, followed by flowers, with woods and resins actually improving with age.

Essential oils are sold in either ounces or milliliters (ml).

¼ ounce = 7.4 ml = approximately 150 to 160 drops = 2 liquid drams

Other close equivalences commonly sold are:

5 ml = ⅙ ounce
10 ml = ⅓ ounce
15 ml = ½ ounce = 4 liquid drams
30 ml = 1 ounce = 8 liquid drams

A standard dropper holds about 20 to 25 drops, which is 1 ml.

Magical Timing

Just as the hourly, yearly (solar), or monthly (lunar) cycle at which the plant raw materials are harvested makes a difference in the quality and potency of the essential oil, so too is timing important when making and consecrating your tarot oils. Magical work, to be at its most effective, operates by cycles of the sun, moon, and planets. Each day, and hour of the day, is dedicated to a particular planetary (and thence divine) energy.

Use the following "Table of Planetary 'Hours'" if you wish to take planetary influences into account when making your tarot oils. To use the table, you must calculate the "hours" as follows: from newspapers or astrological calendars that publish the times of sunrise and sunset, determine the total number of hours of daylight and divide by twelve, which yields the daylight planetary "hour." This "hour" will be slightly more or less than a sixty-minute hour (equaling it only during the seasonal equinoxes, the times of equal daylight and darkness). Follow the same procedure to find the nighttime planetary "hour," whose length will be different from the daylight "hour." In the following table, the first through twelfth "hours" are the daylight "hours," and thirteenth through twenty-fourth are the nighttime "hours."

I suggest that you charge and make your oils, then wait at least three days before consecrating them (so that the molecules can begin to blend), but this is not absolutely necessary. You can also increase the magical forces involved by making each oil on a day and time that is appropriate to its individual astrological energies, then consecrating an entire set on a day when the astrological energies are at a desired peak. Alternatively, make the oils on the new moon and charge them on the full moon. Above all, go with your own needs and intuitions.

The season of the year in which you make and use your oils can also be chosen for its symbolic significance, for instance, a sun oil made at either the summer or winter solstice.

TABLE OF PLANETARY "HOURS"

The 1st "hour" begins at sunrise and each "hour" is added from that moment.

"HOUR"	SUN Sunday	MOON Monday	MARS Tuesday	MERCURY Wednesday	JUPITER Thursday	VENUS Friday	SATURN Saturday
1st	Sun	Moon	Mars	Mercury	Jupiter	Venus	Saturn
2nd	Venus	Saturn	Sun	Moon	Mars	Mercury	Jupiter
3rd	Mercury	Jupiter	Venus	Saturn	Sun	Moon	Mars
4th	Moon	Mars	Mercury	Jupiter	Venus	Saturn	Sun
5th	Saturn	Sun	Moon	Mars	Mercury	Jupiter	Venus
6th	Jupiter	Venus	Saturn	Sun	Moon	Mars	Mercury
7th	Mars	Mercury	Jupiter	Venus	Saturn	Sun	Moon
8th	Sun	Moon	Mars	Mercury	Jupiter	Venus	Saturn
9th	Venus	Saturn	Sun	Moon	Mars	Mercury	Jupiter
10th	Mercury	Jupiter	Venus	Saturn	Sun	Moon	Mars
11th	Moon	Mars	Mercury	Jupiter	Venus	Saturn	Sun
12th	Saturn	Sun	Moon	Mars	Mercury	Jupiter	Venus
13th	Jupiter	Venus	Saturn	Sun	Moon	Mars	Mercury
14th	Mars	Mercury	Jupiter	Venus	Saturn	Sun	Moon
15th	Sun	Moon	Mars	Mercury	Jupiter	Venus	Saturn
16th	Venus	Saturn	Sun	Moon	Mars	Mercury	Jupiter
17th	Mercury	Jupiter	Venus	Saturn	Sun	Moon	Mars
18th	Moon	Mars	Mercury	Jupiter	Venus	Saturn	Sun
19th	Saturn	Sun	Moon	Mars	Mercury	Jupiter	Venus
20th	Jupiter	Venus	Saturn	Sun	Moon	Mars	Mercury
21st	Mars	Mercury	Jupiter	Venus	Saturn	Sun	Moon
22nd	Sun	Moon	Mars	Mercury	Jupiter	Venus	Saturn
23rd	Venus	Saturn	Sun	Moon	Mars	Mercury	Jupiter
24th	Mercury	Jupiter	Venus	Saturn	Sun	Moon	Mars

Tarot Oil Techniques

Steps for Charging and Making Tarot Oils

Although tarot oils will work without any ceremony, I find that dedicating the oils while you make them, consecrating them once they are made, consciously setting intentions when you use them, then ritually anointing yourself will intensify your experience with the oils. Use the suggestions below or create your own rituals. The important thing is to not only look at your materials and say the words but also to imagine (and eventually experience) the actual flow and transformation of energies.

Basically, you want the oils to take on the most spiritual characteristics of each corresponding tarot card. You want to invite into the oil the essential energy of these archetypal forces, so that the spiritual entities drawn to you will work toward your greatest good. You want the oils to be alive—not only with their own life forces and healing qualities but also with their angelic and magical powers of transformation. When making the oils, do so with intention, envisioning your purpose clearly. Try to sense the movement and building of energies. These awarenesses will become stronger the more you work with them.

1. Prepare everything you need:

   - clean bottles

   - oils (essential and carrier)

   - a small funnel or a measuring cup with pointed spout for pouring the carrier oil

   - one or more eyedroppers (or you may pour your oils drop by drop from the bottle)

   - alcohol and paper towels for cleanups

   - labels and pen

   - the tarot deck of your choice

   - an auspicious day or time as mentioned above, if desired.

2. Take out the Major Arcana tarot card for the oil you want to make. Place it behind or near your work area so you can see it clearly—but where it won't get oil on it.

3. Clear the energy from your workplace with a natural incense. I prefer burning dried sage or cedar in a seashell and wafting the smoke with a feather over the bottles, the cards, and over and around myself. Always open a door or window to allow egress for energies you don't want. If you wish, call on the four directions and formally create your sacred space.

4. Relax and ground yourself (see "Grounding and Centering Process" on page 132) and state your intention clearly. With your arms extended, palms out, breathe through your hands until they seem to pump with radiant light. With your hands thus sensitized, pick up each oil and ask its spiritual essence if it is truly appropriate to your task. I suggest you write down the response you receive in a journal reserved for your tarot work. You can also use a pendulum or muscle-testing to confirm my suggestions or your own choice of oils for each tarot card.

5. Pour your carrier oil into your bottle while acknowledging its source.

6. Take your chosen essential oil in your hand. Look at the tarot card and evoke in your mind the symbols and qualities of that card. Become aware of how they correspond to the natural characteristics of the essential oil you hold. Close your eyes and imagine the card as fully as possible (open your eyes and check for additional details and then imagine the scene again until it is absolutely clear in your mind's eye). Now dedicate the oil to its forthcoming use, saying something like the following general dedication (or be more specific by mentioning specific qualities of the card):

I bless you and dedicate you to my purpose of coming to know and understand myself and my place both on this planet and in the world of Spirit through the workings of [name the tarot card here].

Tarot Oil Techniques   141

Then carefully pour the essential oil into your bottle of carrier oil, drop by drop (or use a clean eye dropper). If there is more than one essential oil, then repeat this step for each oil.

7. Put the cap on your bottle and acknowledge that these energies are now encapsulated therein. Shake the bottle (or tap it firmly against your palm) and see the disparate forces begin to blend and harmonize into one. Label the bottle!

8. Thank those beings who have been invoked or drawn to your working, release the directions (if invoked), and open your sacred circle.

The Egyptians and many other peoples accompanied the making of oils and incense with the reading of sacred books. You might want to play meditation music (Tibetan bells or nature sounds) or begin and end your session with a taped journey to a sacred space.

Consecrating Your Tarot Oils

After your tarot oils are made, you will want to consecrate them (see the comments on timing for recommendations on when to do this).

In front of each bottle (or under each bottle if there is absolutely no oil on the outside of the bottles), place the corresponding tarot card from the Major Arcana of the deck you most like working with. Again you may use incense to clear the energy around the bottles and cards and to help you clarify and focus your intent.

If you wish, call on the four directions. Ground your energy again, as in the previous process. Breathe in the energy from earth and sky—from the rich soils and underground rivers beneath you, all the green and growing things on the surface of the earth, and from the light of the sun and moon and stars above you. Breathe out your intention through the pure filter of your heart, down your arms and through the palms of your hands, so that it will go into the bottles of oil before you. Imagine your intention as carried on light rays of an appropriate color—ask your higher self for guidance or envision white or gold light.

Invoke whatever spirits, gods, or goddesses you want present to witness or infuse your work. Write or spontaneously speak your own words that will best charge your oils to your purpose. Or you can use the charge given here:

> *May these oils be here blessed,*
> *So that the ancient wisdom and gifts*
> *of the archetypes of the tarot*
> *can enter into them now.*
> *And so that I, and all others who use them,*
> *may partake of both the life force*
> *of the plants of the earth for growth and healing,*
> *and of the power and knowledge*
> *of the 22 tarot keys for opening the gates to Spirit*
> *for my good and for the greatest good of all.*
> *May these oils be always used with wisdom and understanding,*
> *drawing from both mercy and severity,*
> *guiding me to walk in beauty.*
> *That thus I may achieve victory and splendor*
> *within my own foundation, and*
> *manifest the crown of spirit in the kingdom of this world.*
> *So mote it be.*

In the spirit and innocence of the Fool, inhale deeply, then blow that Spirit-breath over the oils, pouring your intentions from your hands into the oils at the same time.

Anointing Yourself with Oil

There are several reasons for anointing yourself with aromatic oils:

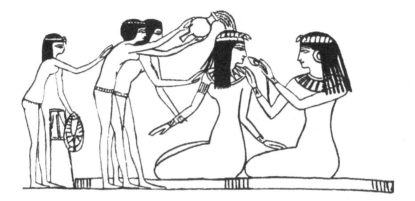

1. It takes you out of normal space and time, raising your vibrations so that you can receive the astral forces.
2. It creates an "aura of protection," shielding you from energies you don't want.
3. It then acts as a magnet, attracting to you the energies related to the oil and symbols with which you are working.
4. It also strengthens the corresponding spirits or energies so that they can manifest into the physical world. This is especially good for any rituals where you are taking on a "god form"; that is, allowing that divine force to work through you.

Take the oil of your choice, open the bottle, and as the aroma arises, visualize the presence of the tarot archetype that corresponds to it. Affirm the qualities you want to access from the oil. If you are simply exploring the qualities and effects of the oils, you may want to ask something like: "What do I most need to learn from you (today)?"

Put some oil on your fingers and in a counterclockwise direction (to go inward) or vertically down (to bring from spirit into manifestation), etc., rub the oil on significant parts of your body. For instance, rub oil on one or more chakras, envisioning how you want each to be affected. You can also anoint yourself on your hands and feet, ears, genitals, or wherever, while being careful not to get oils on mucus membranes or in your eyes. Say out loud, as you anoint your throat, for example, what you would like to have happen: "May this oil help me speak my truth clearly."

Examples of Intentions Relating to the Chakras

- The *crown of your head*—for opening to spirit.

- Your *third eye*—for seeing clearly.

- Your *throat*—for speaking truthfully without holding back.

- Your *heart*—for actions that come from love or for balance.

- Your *solar plexus*—for focusing your will and power.

- Your *spleen/belly*—for accessing your deepest emotions; and for women, your womb wisdom.

- The *base of your spine*—for grounding and getting to the root of the matter.

You can also anoint:

- The *base of your skull*—for accessing instinct, memories, or past lives.

- Along your *backbone*—specifically for back issues, to help you carry on or uphold a value.

- Your *hands*—to consecrate whatever you are handling or passing on and to give meaning to everything you do.

Tarot Oil Techniques

- Your *feet*—for walking the path of your intention. (Note: deeply massaging your feet with tarot massage oil allows you to access all of yourself through the meridians in a practical way—see any diagram on foot reflexology for more information.)

- Your *genitals*—for sacred sexuality. (Caution: do not put directly on mucous membranes unless directed by a knowledgeable aromatherapist.)

- The *seat of your senses*, such as *around* but not in your eyes, ears, nose, mouth, and fingers so as to open and attune them to higher vibrations. (Be very careful not to let the oil get too near your eyes!)

- Any *other pulse points* (like neck and wrist)—for connecting with the flow of heart-blood through your body and attuning to your personal energy expression.

You may, of course, anoint someone else with these oils—especially in rituals of blessing, welcoming, bonding, or allocating (passing on a force). Remember that only the persons themselves can dedicate themselves, but you may bless them or acknowledge some quality you see.

Uses for the Tarot Oils

Use common sense when applying tarot and aromatherapy oils. Don't anoint yourself with Moon oil (18) and expect to do well at a job requiring concentration and precision; you may find yourself fantasizing and daydreaming instead. And don't put on Tower oil (16) for an evening of gentle romance and quiet "sharing," which could be shattered by aggressive feelings and intense sexual response. Of course, if that is what you want, go for it!

Shaykh Hakim Moinuddin Chishti in *The Book of Sufi Healing* suggests that when a mental or emotional condition is being treated, put one drop of oil on a small bit of cotton and place it on the ridge *above* the opening of the *right* ear (not inside the ear itself). This is an important acupuncture point where five cranial nerves come together to form a ganglion.[3] This is best done as part of a deep meditation or when you can rest or relax (depending on the oil and your intention), for the effect can be immediate and pronounced. I have found that it is often accompanied by a heightening of the senses, including an impression of taste, but can lead to a headache if not done with care. It is an excellent way to test the effects of an oil—if you quiet yourself and "listen" carefully to your bodily responses. Use this technique for meditations or channeling when you want to communicate with an oil.

Bearing these thoughts in mind, try the following techniques.

Tarot Meditations

Work your way through the Major Arcana in order, focusing successively on each card and the corresponding tarot oil. Do this at your own pace, per day or per week, for study and contemplation. Use the oil to help you align with that energy and to keep your focus in your meditation. Whenever you notice the aroma, note how your thoughts or activities at that moment are related to the card. Keep a journal of your explorations.

Daily Card Divination

Draw one Major Arcana card per day, at random, to represent what you need to learn from the events of the day. Use the oil to remind you of the energy that you are accessing and learning from, and as you smell it through the day, note what is happening around you that may be connected with that card or the message it may have for you.

Daily Oil Divination

Closing your eyes, select a tarot oil at random. Without looking to see which it is, anoint yourself and then observe the day's events and people's reactions to you. At the end of the day, identify the oil you used. After a while, you will know the scents immediately and which cards they go with, but until then, this is an interesting way to discover their effects for yourself without preconceived judgements.

Moving Meditations

Anoint yourself and then do a moving meditation, many of which can be found online. Let the aroma move you through the landscape of the card.

Lifetime and Year Cards

Determine those cards (based on your full birth date) that most closely represent your personality and soul purpose or your card for the year (based on your birth month and day, plus the current year)—see appendix A. Use the oil when you meditate on these cards or to dialogue with a figure on the card. Refer to my books *Tarot for Your Self: A Workbook for the Inward Journey* or *Archetypal Tarot: What Your Birth Card Reveals about Your Personality, Your Path, and Your Potential* for more information on determining and working with these special, personal cards.

Special Tasks

Select a tarot oil that will prepare you for a special task. Anoint yourself with that oil. For instance, when going to court or negotiating contracts, use Justice (11). To release someone or something with love, use Death (13). For open communications, you could use either The Lovers (6) or The Magician (1).

Altars and Candles

Use tarot oils for anointing objects for your personal altar or for "dressing" a candle. Such a "dressing" or anointing magnetizes the candle and impresses it with your intention. To do so, ground and center. Set your intention. Find the center of the candle. Place a small amount of oil in your hands and rub them together until warm. With the exposed wick upright, grasp the candle on either side of the center. With your right hand, stroke up toward the wick (called the north pole). Then, with your left hand, stroke from the center toward the bottom (called the south pole). Continue stroking alternate ends until you feel a magnetism build up within the candle. Use this in candle-magic rituals.[4] Anoint a letter or spellbook with a selected tarot oil to add that intent to it. If you use undiluted essential oils, they will not leave an oily mark on paper. Objects anointed like this should not be taken lightly: treat them with respect, for they contain the power of your intention.

Dream Incubation

Incubate a dream with a tarot oil. Place 2 or 3 drops of oil on a piece of cotton and put it under your head when you sleep. Use an oil associated with dreaming (such as The Moon [18], The High Priestess [2], or The Hanged Man [12]) or one for astral traveling (such as The Chariot [7] or The World [21]). Or use one like Strength (8) that has rosemary for making your dream memory strong. Experiment with the kind of dreams each one will give you.

Making Affirmations

At the conclusion of any tarot reading, choose the card that most specifically expresses the qualities you want to develop in yourself (or your client when doing a professional reading; see below) as a result of the events described in the reading. Describe those qualities based on what you see in the card, then turn those statements into an affirmation to be said as you anoint yourself (or your client) with the corresponding oil. The affirmation should be said daily and accompanied by the scent. Eventually the scent itself will evoke the qualities of that affirmation in you.

The appropriate card is usually present in the reading, but if a Minor Arcana card was selected, you may use that specific oil or the Major Arcana tarot oil that most closely corresponds. Information on creating affirmations and temporarily charging a tarot oil with a specific affirmation appears on page 152.

Tarot Oil Techniques

Professional Tarot Readings

Use the "Making Affirmations" section above to complete every professional reading. Your client will remember the reading with extraordinary clarity for hours afterward, and they will leave feeling positive and uplifted and have a direction for growth and a goal by which to gauge future decisions. Make sure it is the client and not you, the reader, who picks the card and states the qualities they want to develop. As reader, you should write down the client's statements and then help them formulate those qualities into an affirmation. (It is important to use only the client's own words!) Clients can then anoint themselves with a tarot oil, or you can put several drops of essential oil on a tissue or small square of heavy watercolor paper that they can smell whenever saying their affirmation. (If wrapped in plastic, it should hold the scent for one or two weeks.)

Before Reading for Others

Anoint yourself in order to be able to channel the highest and clearest truth to the querent. What Major Arcana archetype do you want to access as a reader? High Priestess, Hermit, Star, Hierophant, Magician, Temperance? What energy do you want to speak from? Go light on the scent, as some clients may be overly sensitive to aromas.

Tarot Classes

Teachers of tarot can use the oils in classes, along with colors, sounds, and movement to create a complete tarot environment for the study of each card. Again, be sensitive to their needs.

Groups

Where groups of people meet on a regular basis, such as for seasonal rituals or classes, you can use scents to quickly link the people together and to give them a group identity. This spiritual group energy/entity is called an egregore.

Talismans

Make a *talisman* out of a piece of cotton or linen rag paper (heavy watercolor paper is excellent). Go through the tarot deck to pick out cards that most represent what you want to create. Anoint the talisman paper with full-strength essential oils as you meditate on your purpose. Create an affirmation that states that you have achieved that purpose. Once the oil has set, draw symbols on the talisman, as suggested by the tarot card's correspondences (see the "Table of Tarot Correspondences" on page 42) and from your affirmation. Place the talisman in a small cloth bag and wear it around your neck.

Channeled Readings

You can use this process to do "channeled" readings or as a classroom exercise for attunement with the tarot.[5] While the designated querent or "readee" thinks of a question, you, the reader, ask what archetypal energy can best respond; then, from a face-down deck, draw a Major Arcana card. *Anoint yourself with the related tarot oil.* Close your eyes, ground, and ask for the presence of your guides or higher self. Imagine the card in all its details, opening your eyes once or twice to check the card until you can see every detail in your mind's eye. Imagine the card getting larger and larger until you can step over the border and into the environment of the card. Asking permission first, step backward into the image of the central figure on the card, shifting your energy until you get an exact fit.

You have now taken on the "valence" of that tarot archetype. Let the readee know when you are ready so that they can ask their question. Respond from the perspective of the tarot archetype. Let both the scent and the feeling of "being" that archetype dictate the response. When you have finished dialoguing about the question, you should step out of the archetype, turn and thank it for its assistance, then step over the edge of the card; see it grow smaller until you feel yourself sitting back in the room where you began. Ground your energy. If you are trading readings, switch roles at this point.

Tarot Oil Techniques

Using Affirmations with Tarot Oils

Creating a Personal Affirmation

Affirmations are positive statements that create openings—literally and figuratively—in the walls around us. On the other hand, negations (no matter how helpful they sound) only create greater enclosure and imprisonment.

1. To create an affirmation, first determine the qualities you want to develop in yourself. Look at the related tarot card, or read about the essential oils, to help you generate specific, concrete statements. Write down key words and phrases, affirming that you now have those qualities.

2. *Always use first person, present tense.* Never say "I will . . . ," as that puts your statement forever in the future. Try turning one of the descriptive words into an active verb that shows you *doing* something, like, "I trust," or "I dance," or "I construct."

3. Whenever you say "no," "not," "un-," "never," or any other negative, rephrase your statement. For instance, if you say "I am no longer afraid of the dark," ask yourself what quality would demonstrate that. If you "are not afraid," then what are you? Perhaps you might say, "I find security and comfort in the dark," or "I face the dark with trust and belief in myself." Note how different these last two statements are from the original negative statement.

4. Check your affirmation by saying it out loud three times. Do you sound convinced, vital, and empowered? Does it ring true? Modify your affirmation until it "resonates" right.[6]

Charging a Tarot Oil with Your Affirmation

Take out the oil corresponding to your affirmation and, if you wish, the tarot card itself. If it is The High Priestess, for instance, be sure that you can see her image clearly in your mind. Center and ground yourself; often just one or two conscious, deep breaths will do. Open the bottle of oil. Acknowledge the presence of the High Priestess energy within the oil. Inhale the High Priestess energy, associating the scent with both the words and content of your affirmation. When you sense that the connection is made, speak your affirmation over the oil three times. (For example, *"I act from my inner wisdom and deepest knowledge."*) Now breathe out the qualities of the High Priestess. Anoint yourself with the oil and feel her presence. Finally, say your affirmation three times out loud, firmly and with expression. Be aware that other qualities of the High Priestess, which you have not named (and may not even be aware of), will also be present—for you are working with an archetype of vast numinous energy! So ask that the effects of this work be always for your greatest good and that of all other beings.

Using Your Affirmation

Write your affirmation on an index card and tape it to your bathroom mirror. Every morning, anoint yourself with the corresponding tarot oil, look yourself in the eyes in the mirror, and say your affirmation out loud three times. You should do this daily for at least twenty-one days (three weeks), then give it a rest. Say your affirmation during the day whenever you want. Use the scent of the essential oil to remind you of your purpose.

When you make decisions that are not in accordance with your affirmation, don't give them energy by becoming angry or upset. With gentle compassion and humor, thank the situation for letting you recognize your "stuck" places. On the other hand, when you make a decision that accords with your affirmation, pat yourself on the back and give yourself a small, symbolic reward (a fresh rose, a gold star, a long bath with essential oils).

Ritual Uses for Tarot Cards and Oils

Use the Major Arcana tarot cards and their related essential oils in rituals, meditations, and processes for the purposes suggested below. Lay your chosen cards out in front of you to symbolize what you want to create. Remember that anointing yourself with any oil will bring out those qualities in yourself. For example, the High Priestess oil will bring out the High Priestess in yourself and can be used whenever you assume that role in a ceremony.

The Fool

For travel, spontaneity and excitement, openness and trust, getting in touch with your inner child, taking a leap of faith.

The Magician

For writing, communicating, conjuring and creating illusion, cunning, craft and skills, channeling and moving power, focusing, cultivating change, individuality, self-initiation, magical wisdom.

The High Priestess

For past-life meditation; menstruation and menopause; calmness and serenity; being whole unto yourself (not belonging to another); drawing down the moon; emotional objectivity and balance; creating an ebb and flow; receptivity to tides and cycles, psychic knowledge, and inner wisdom.

The Empress

For love, fertility, relating, creativity, nurturing, harmonizing and integrating, aesthetic and sensual pleasure, mother or mothering issues, pregnancy and birthing, creating beauty,[7] emotional security, work in nature.

The Emperor

For building, starting new projects, organizing, establishing authority, making rules and laws, father or fathering issues, career, creating new directions.

The Hierophant (or The High Priest)

For teaching and learning, public speaking, advising and wise counsel, issues with large organizations or cultural/religious institutions, grounding, practical applications of abstract ideas.

The Lovers

For relationship and communication issues, making choices, balancing masculine and feminine energies, marriages and commitments, responding to love or inspiration, Tantric rituals.

The Chariot

For traveling, protection and shielding, directing energy outward, drive and ambition, assertiveness, mastery and temporary success, focus on a goal, controlling emotions or opposing forces.

Strength

For life-force energy, general health and vitality, self-expression, handling anger and rage, coming from the heart, alignment with nature, connecting with animals, menstrual rituals, enchanting and bewitching wild things, facing your fears, endurance, forging strong bonds.

The Hermit

For spiritual quests and journeys, patience, standing alone, teaching and guidance, completing things, reviewing your life and self-contemplation, remembering your past in preparation for the future.

The Wheel of Fortune

For change, transformation, attunement with the seasons, creating a sacred circle, expanding opportunities, spreading messages and wide communications, general luck and good fortune.

Tarot Oil Techniques

Justice

For being true to yourself, legal and money matters, fair and just contractual agreements, negotiating, evaluating, clear thinking and truthfulness, balancing, awareness of the three-fold law of return. (Place between two other cards to show them in balance.)

The Hanged Man

For sacrificing and surrendering, mystical visions, dreams, inducing altered states, acknowledging pain and loss, releasing emotional cords to others, reversing old patterns, turning things around, looking at addiction and scapegoating patterns.

Death

For easing transitions, releasing, dying, pruning, letting go, cutting off, getting down to the most elemental skeletal support of your being, sexual release, dying to the state of separateness and being born into union with the All.

Temperance

For rebirth, general healing, angelic guidance, blending and combining energies (place between two other cards to represent what you are blending), alchemical transformations, compassion, balancing chakras and auras.

The Devil

For increasing sexual energy, mirth, play, bedevilment, facing your fears, shadow work or play, setting wards or guarding, material world matters, power and achievement. (This card is dangerous to use for power or control over others.)

The Tower

For burning up, exploding, breaking down or through obstacles, opening things up, raising energy or the cone of power, generating, renovating, sexual potency, fertility. It can be dangerous to use in a way that hurts others, whether through anger or righteously felt cancel-culture activities.

The Star

For reconsecrating the body after abusive situations, cleansing, purifying and renewing, self-esteem, liberating, meditating, linking with the universe, web activities, ecological and astrological workings, hope, faith.

The Moon

For astral traveling, dreamwork, receptivity, acceptance, sleeping, pulling or drawing out, evolution and cellular change, facing your fears, past-life or ancestor work, hiding things, alignment with lunar cycles, moon magic.

The Sun

For birthing, marriages, healing, good health and vitality, success, prosperity, fame, recognition, finding things, enlightenment, warmth, inner-child work.

Judgment

For final decisions, critical perception and good judgment, transitions and major transformations, sending out a call, awakening to purpose, commitment to a cause, workings that involve society's collective experiences and social media.

The World

For shielding, grounding, creating an aura of protection, dancing, integration; establishing boundaries, form, or sacred space; recreating oneself, traveling through the cosmos, success, wholeness, completion, experiencing your multidimensional self.

Tarot Oil Techniques

CHAPTER 8

Tarot Spreads

The Quintessence Spread

This spread is about the quintessential meaning of your current actions—that is, their most concentrated nature or expression. The fifth essence, in relation to the traditional four of fire, earth, air, and water, expresses what is left after these physical elements have done their work. Just as essential oils represent the soul, the divine within the physical, so too does the fifth card in this spread. Determine how the elements themselves are functioning within you by interpreting the first four cards. The balance of your elemental energies is indicated by which elements appear the most, especially in their own position, where they function at their best. For instance, if there are three Wand cards in the spread, your fiery energy is strong.

But if none of these Wands appears in the Fire position, you might be using this energy unconsciously or inappropriately.

Interpret a card in each of the elemental positions by thinking of what happens when the elements mix naturally. When a Cups card (Water) is in the Earth position, think of mixing dirt and water. Mud? Or water in a canal? Reflect back on how this would modify the meaning of the card. For instance, the 2 of Cups in the Earth position might indicate that the relationship pictured on the card was well channeled or so stable that it was practically "stuck in the mud."

- Keeping all cards upright (no reversals), shuffle them and spread them face down in a fan. Select a card for the Fire within you and place it to the South. Select a card for the Water within you and place it to the West. Select a card for the Air within you and place it to the East. Select a card for the Earth within you and place it to the North. You now have four cards before you. Leave a space in the center for a fifth card, to be selected in a moment.

- Interpret the cards based on the questions given below. Then select your Quintessence card as follows.

- Add together the numbers on each of the cards. People cards and The Fool have no number! Reduce the total to 22 or below. For instance, if you drew the Queen of Cups, the 6 of Wands, Temperance, and The Fool, you would add $0 + 6 + 14 + 0 = 20$. Place the Major Arcana card of the corresponding number (20 = Judgement)—even if it already appears in the spread—in the central position. (If your total is 22, then use the Fool as your Quintessence card.) The card in this position is always interpreted in terms of its highest qualities.

Answer these questions in terms of the card you drew in each position. Note: Wands work best in Fire and Air, are neutral in Earth, and are problematic in Water; Swords work best in Air and Fire, are neutral in Water, and are problematic in Earth; Cups work best in Water and Earth, are neutral in Air, and are problematic in Fire; Pentacles work best in Earth and Water, are neutral in Fire, and are problematic in Air. "Problematic" means that their expression might be somewhat blocked, unconscious, or expressed inappropriately.

POSITION 1 = FIRE
What is inspiring me and getting me fired up? How am I expressing my passions?

POSITION 2 = WATER
How do I feel about what's happening? What is my emotional reaction?

POSITION 3 = AIR
What am I thinking about? How am I organizing or defending matters?

POSITION 4 = EARTH
What am I manifesting? How am I trying to establish self-worth?

POSITION 5 = THE QUINTESSENCE
This card represents the true value of what you can create at this time. It is your soul-expression that is trying to come out through the energies and actions pictured by the surrounding cards. It is a magnetic force drawing you to the center of your being. This card answers the questions: How can I triumph? What energy within me can bring the four different aspects described by the other cards into harmonious balance? What is the highest quality in myself that is trying to be expressed?

Use your answers to these questions to create a personal affirmation. Charge the corresponding tarot oil with that affirmation and use it as suggested in the section called "Creating a Personal Affirmation" on page 152.

The Creative Work-Cycle Spread

Use this spread when planning rituals or involved in any creative project.

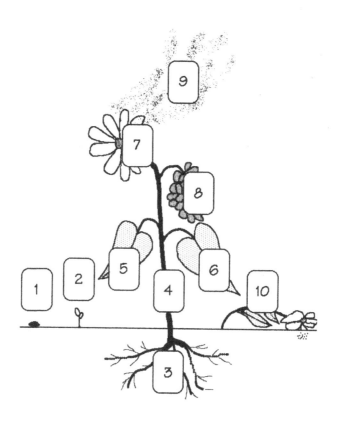

1. Seed = What is your seed intent?

2. Sprout = What is the challenge you must meet in order to get started or continue?

3. Root = Where is this intent rooted in the past? (past lives, previous experience, unconscious patterns and assumptions)

4. Stalk/Trunk = What supports your work?

5 & 6. What are your choices or options for creative action? If necessary, you can add more leaves to represent alternative options.

7. Blossom = What are you expressing or putting out to the world? (This card may indicate whether your work will draw or repel others. Is this appropriate to the intent of your work?)

8. Fruit = What will be the material result of this work?

9. Fragrance = What is the spiritual import or lesson of this work?

10. The Decayed Plant and Dried Seed = What must you release to create room for transformation and new life?

The Magic Spread

Use this spread for creating your own reality.

1. Use whatever spread you most employ for your own readings. The Celtic Cross spread, for instance, works quite well. Familiarity with the spread adds to its effectiveness.

2. Go through the deck with the pictures face up and select a card for each position that shows you already having, doing, and being what you want to create.

3. Be as specific and concrete as possible in describing why you are putting each card in each position. For instance, "The Six of Pentacles in the Near Future position shows me receiving royalties for my book. The six indicates they will reach six figures."

4. Go through the spread as if it were a reading. Look up meanings, even if you don't usually need to do so. Make any changes necessary. Then write up your interpretation as if it were happening to you right now. You have become what the spread describes.

5. Determine one card from the spread that best expresses the qualities you most want to develop in yourself. Refer to the section on creating an affirmation in the previous chapter, and use your affirmation with the corresponding tarot oil daily.

Do not do this spread for someone who is not present, and do not do it about other people. In other words, don't do a spread in which Mrs. Johnson changes her mind and decides to hire you as scriptwriter for the new comedy series because your competitor suddenly took ill. This sort of magic is asking for trouble, because the three-fold law of return will send it back to you magnified three times—you may lose the job as suddenly as you gained it. Instead, do a spread in which you are happily and creatively working as a comedy scriptwriter and receiving ample compensation and recognition for your work. For love magic, concentrate on the qualities you need in yourself in order to draw the perfect person for the kind of relationship you most want. Describe in cards the *characteristics* of a person you think will satisfy your needs, but let the universe provide the person rather than trying to force someone specific into that picture.

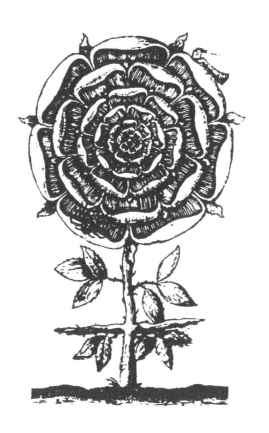

APPENDIX A

The Lifetime and Year Cards

Note: The following material is adapted from *Archetypal Tarot: What Your Birth Card Reveals about Your Personality, Your Path, and Your Potential* by Mary K. Greer (Weiser Books, 2021). Refer to this book for detailed information about the tarot constellations.

Based on your date of birth, you have specific tarot cards, known as the lifetime cards, that form your "pattern of personal destiny." Using your birthdate, let's numerologically calculate your personality, soul, hidden factor/teacher, and year cards.

The Personality and Soul Cards

First, to find your personality/soul combination (your pattern of personal destiny), add together your month, day, and year of birth—like this:

For example:

Margaret Mead (famous anthropologist)
December 16, 1901 = 12
16
1901
1929

Then, add each digit in the resulting number: 1 + 9 + 2 + 9 = 21. *Keep any number from 1 to 22.* The resulting personality number indicates the personality card, which in this case is 21, corresponding to the twenty-first Major Arcana card: The World (21). *Your personality card indicates personality characteristics that you develop easily and lessons that you learn early in your life, as they seem to resonate with your essential nature.*

Then add together 2 + 1 = 3 to find the soul number. Anthropologist Margaret Mead's soul number (3) indicates a soul card that corresponds to the third Major Arcana card, The Empress (3). *Your soul card shows your soul purpose: those qualities in yourself that you must express and use in order to feel fulfilled in whatever you do.*

In some cases, the number will add up to more than 22. Since there are only 22 Major Arcana cards, reduce the number to 22 or less.

For example:

Mick Jagger (singer, musician)
July 26, 1943 = 07
                26
               1943
               ————
               1976 = 1 + 9 + 7 + 6 = 23
               2 + 3 = 5 = Hierophant

In the case of musician Mick Jagger, the fifth card, The Hierophant, is both his personality and soul card. Anyone with the same number for both cards is specifically working on their soul purpose in this lifetime. It makes the person more focused and directed.

If the reduced sum of your month, day, plus year is 19, there will be three cards.

The Lifetime and Year Cards

For example:

Martin Luther King, Jr. (reverend and civil rights activist)
January 15, 1929 = 1

$$15$$
$$\underline{1929}$$
$$1945 = 1 + 9 + 4 + 5 = 19$$
$$1 + 9 = 10$$
$$1 + 0 = 1$$

It is only when your birthdate totals 19, like that of Martin Luther King above, that you will have such a triple sequence. In some ways all three cards defy categories, but, for your use here, you can consider The Sun (19) as your personality card, The Magician (1) as your soul card, and The Wheel of Fortune (10) as your teacher card (more about the teacher card later). People with this sequence must learn to communicate their individual creative expression. Their personal identity and sense of self will be inextricably combined with their life and soul purpose. Their ability to relate to others will depend on a harmony of vision and sense of shared purpose.

If your birthdate adds up to 22, you combine great impulsiveness and great mastery, a fine line to balance. The number 22 represents 0 (The Fool), since there are 22 cards in the Major Arcana, and 22 in numerology is a master number signifying great wisdom or great folly. It reduces to 4 (The Emperor). Bill Gates, founder of Microsoft, born on October 28, 1955, is an example of a 22-4 personality.

Determining Your Personality and Soul Cards

Add: The month you were born: _____

The day you were born: _____

The year you were born: _____

Equals: _____

Add each digit in that sum:

_____ + _____ + _____ + _____ = _____

If you have a double-digit answer, add again:

_____ + _____ = _____

My personality number is _____ (the higher of two numbers if 22 or less).

The Major Arcana card corresponding to this number is:

_____

Personality Card

My soul number is ____ (the single-digit number in your final reduction).

The Major Arcana card corresponding to this number is:

_____

Soul Card

The Hidden Factor Card

In addition to the numbers obtained directly through addition and reduction, there is frequently another number-and-card concept indirectly connected with your birthdate that I call your hidden factor (or teacher) card. The chart on page 170 will help you determine this number.

Tarot Constellations

A "tarot constellation" consists of all the cards with the *same prime number* (1 through 9), as well as all the other Major Arcana cards whose numbers reduce to that prime number. Their energies constellate, or come together, based on similar principles; that is, on vibrational essences of like quality.

Let's go back to the first birthdate used as an example, that of Margaret Mead: her personality card is The World (21) and her soul card is The Empress (3). By combining these numbers, we are able to refer to her as a

The Lifetime and Year Cards

"21-3." Now look at the "Patterns of Personal Destiny" chart and notice that there is one other Major Arcana number listed in her constellation: 12. Since she did not get a 12 in her calculations, it is a hidden aspect of her birth vibrational essence. This is her hidden factor card: The Hanged Man (12). All the 3s of the Minor Arcana also belong to her constellation, which is called the constellation of love and creative imagination.

PATTERNS OF PERSONAL DESTINY				
Personality & Soul Card Patterns	Hidden Factor (Teacher) Cards	Minor Arcana Cards	**Constellation** **of the**	Principle of
1-1 10-1 19-10-1	10 & 19 19 10 (Teacher)	10's & 1's	**Magician** (Sun, Wheel of Fortune, Magician)	Will and Focused Consciousness
2-2 11-2 20-2	11 & 20 20 11	2's	**High Priestess** (Judgement, Justice, High Priestess)	Balanced Judgement Through Intuitive Awareness
3-3 12-3 21-3	12 & 21 21 12	3's	**Empress** (World, Hanged One, Empress)	Love and Creative Imagination
4-4 13-4 22-4	13 & 22 22 13	4's	**Emperor** (Fool, Death, Emperor)	Life Force and Realization of Power
5-5 14-5	14 *	5's	**Hierophant** (Temperance, Hierophant)	Teaching and Learning
6-6 15-6	15 *	6's	**Lovers** (Devil, Lovers)	Relatedness and Choice
7-7 16-7	16 *	7's	**Chariot** (Tower, Chariot)	Mastery Through Change
8-8 17-8	17 *	8's	**Strength** (Star, Strength)	Courage and Self-Esteem
9-9	18	9's	**Hermit** (Moon, Hermit)	Introspection and Personal Integrity

Variations

There are three situations in which the hidden factor determination differs from the above:

1. The first variation occurs in constellations 5 through 9, involving the personality-soul patterns 14-5 through 18-9, which contain no hidden factor. For example:

   Marilyn Monroe (Film actress)
   June 1, 1926 = 6

   $$\begin{array}{r} 1 \\ 1926 \\ \hline 1933 = 16 \text{ (Tower)} = \\ 1 + 6 = 7 \text{ (Chariot)} \end{array}$$

   Marilyn Monroe is therefore a 16-7, with The Tower (16) as personality card, and The Chariot (7) as soul card. There is no number not accounted for in her constellation and therefore no hidden factor card. Thus the 16-7 combination—and the 14-5, 15-6, 17-8, and 18-9 combinations—have no hidden factor.

2. The 19-10-1 combination is the second variation. Because The Wheel of Fortune (10) was involved in the computation, it is not "hidden." I call it the teacher card because it does not manifest the "shadow" quality normally associated with the hidden factor card.

3. Lastly, people who are a single 1, 2, 3, or 4 (that is, having personality-soul patterns of 1-1, 2-2, 3-3, or 4-4) have two hidden factor cards, as shown by the chart. For example, a single 4 (or 4-4) has The Fool (22) and Death (13) as hidden factor cards. People with single-card combinations were rare until birthdays began adding up to 2000 to 2007. In fact, there have been no single 1s at all since January 1, 998 CE. The single number of 2 (High Priestess) first appeared for people born on December 31, 1957, but it didn't become frequent until the 1970s and later.

The Lifetime and Year Cards

The Hidden Factor as Shadow Card

Your hidden factor card indicates aspects of yourself that you fear, reject, or don't see, and thus it can also be called the shadow card. The shadow, a term used and defined by Carl Jung, refers to unknown or little-known parts of the personality. They are aspects of ourselves that we deny and thus cannot see directly. However, we remain sensitive to these qualities and therefore tend to see them in others via the psychological mechanism of "projection."

I have found that the hidden factor card acts as your shadow card most strongly during your younger years. The planet Saturn takes twenty-eight to thirty years to complete a circuit of the zodiac; that is, to return to where it was in the sky when you were born. This approximately twenty-nine-year cycle of Saturn is known as your "Saturn return." Thus, Saturn—which represents many of the qualities of your *shadow* and which has much the same significance as the hidden factor—has to face itself every twenty-nine years. By the time they are thirty, most people find that they have learned their greatest lesson from their shadow issues. Carl Jung declared that the *shadow* is your greatest teacher and that only by getting to know your *shadow* can you achieve individuation.

The Hidden Factor Card as Teacher Card

With people over thirty, I tend to call their hidden factor card their teacher card because they are ready to work actively and consciously with its principles.

Your hidden factor card becomes your teacher card when you actively strive to develop and understand its qualities in yourself and in the world around you. Then it represents your strengths.

If you are a 19-10-1, you have no hidden factor card; instead, you have The Wheel of Fortune (10) as your teacher card. In this pattern, you consciously feel that life brings you the experiences you need to achieve your purpose. At worst, you tend to drift through life, never challenged to use your abundant talents.

Determining Your Hidden Factor Card

My hidden factor/teacher number (if you have one) is: _____. The Major Arcana card corresponding to this number is:

Hidden Factor/Teacher Card

The Year Card(s)

For each year of your life, you have a Major Arcana card called the year card. These represent the tests and lessons you experience in any given year. Some Major Arcana cards will appear as your year cards every nine years, while others you will never get. The events that happen to you in any year offer you the opportunity to master new skills and discover more about yourself and your needs. The year card points out what that learning will be about. It indicates the kind of archetypal energies that are constellated in that year, suggesting personal qualities you can work with, such as assertion, compassion, relating, etc. Knowing your year card makes you more aware of the overall situation at your disposal and the kinds of learning opportunities it presents during that year.

Example:

Add the month and date of birth to the current year and reduce it to 22 or less.

Month of birth	12
Day of birth	20
Current year	2025
	2057 = 2 + 0 + 5 + 7 = 14 (Temperance)

In determining the year card, always keep the highest number under 23 and don't reduce it!

The Lifetime and Year Cards

Determining Your Year Card(s)

The month of your birth: _____
The day of your birth: _____
The year in question: _____
Equals: =   _____ (reduce only if 23 or above)
                   =   _____ (year number)

This corresponds to the Major Arcana card:

_____

Year Card

APPENDIX B

Master Chart of the Essential Oils

MASTER CHART OF THE ESSENTIAL OILS			
Essential Oils	Astrological Associations	Major Arcana	Minor Arcana
1 Angelica *Angelica archangelica*	Fire, Sun, Sagittarius.	**Temperance**	—
2 Anise (Aniseed) *Pimpinella anisum*	Air, Mercury, Pluto, Scorpio.	**Judgement**	7 of Pentacles
3 Basil *Ocimum basilicum*	Fire, Mars, Pluto, Scorpio.	**Judgement**	King of Pentacles
4 Bay Laurel *Laurus nobilis*	Fire, Sun, Jupiter, Leo, Aries.	**Emperor**	6 of Wands
5 Bergamot *Citrus bergamia*	Fire, Air, Sun, Jupiter, Sagittarius.	**Temperance**	4 of Swords
6 Black Pepper *Piper nigrum*	Fire, Mars, Aries.	**Tower**	King of Wands

MASTER CHART OF THE ESSENTIAL OILS (continued)

	Essential Oils	Astrological Associations	Major Arcana	Minor Arcana
7	Bois de Rose (Rosewood) *Aniba rosaeodora*	Earth, Venus, Taurus.	**Hierophant**	Queen of Pentacles
8	Camphor *Cinnamomum camphora*	Water, Moon, Cancer.	**High Priestess**	4 of Cups
9	Caraway Seed *Carum carvi*	Air, Earth, Mercury, Virgo.	**Hermit**	Princess of Pentacles
10	Cardamom *Elettaria cardamomum*	Earth, Water, Venus, Taurus.	**Hierophant**	6 of Pentacles
11	Carrot *Daucus carota*	Fire, Water, Sun, Mars, Cancer.	**Chariot**	Prince of Cups
12	Cedar *Cedrus species*	Fire, Sun, Jupiter, Aries, Sagittarius.	**Wheel of Fortune**	9 of Wands
13	Chamomile (Blue) *Matricaria chamomilla*	Air, Water, Uranus, Aquarius.	**Star**	—
14	Chamomile (Roman) *Anthemis nobilis, A. mixta.*	Water, Moon, Cancer.	**Chariot**	Ace of Cups
15	Cinnamon (or Cassia) *Cinnamomum zeylanicum (C. cassia)*	Fire, Sun, Leo.	**Sun**	Ace of Wands
16	Clary Sage *Salvia scalarea*	Earth, Air, Mercury, Saturn, Virgo, Capricorn, Aquarius.	**Devil**	10 of Pentacles
17	Clove *Syzygium aromaticum*	Fire, Jupiter, Sagittarius.	**Wheel of Fortune**	8 of Swords
18	Coriander *Coriandrum sativum*	Fire, Water, Mars, Scorpio.	**Chariot**	8 of Cups
19	Cumin *Cuminum cyminum*	Water, Fire, Mars, Scorpio.	**Death**	—
20	Cypress *Cupressus sempervirens*	Water, Earth, Venus, Saturn, Pluto, Libra, Scorpio.	**Death**	8 of Swords
21	Dill *Anethum graveolens*	Air, Mercury, Gemini.	**Magician**	Prince of Swords
22	Eucalyptus *Eucalyptus globulus*	Air, Mercury, Saturn, Uranus, Gemini, Aquarius.	**Star**	8 of Swords

MASTER CHART OF THE ESSENTIAL OILS (continued)

	Essential Oils	Astrological Associations	Major Arcana	Minor Arcana
23	Fennel *Foeniculum vulgare*	Air, Mercury, Uranus, Gemini, Aquarius.	**Fool**	—
24	Fir *Abies balsamea*	Air, Saturn, Aquarius.	**Star**	King of Swords
25	Frankincense (Olibanum) *Boswellia carterii, B. sacra*	Fire, Sun, Aries, Leo.	**Sun**	3 of Wands
26	Geranium *Pelargonium graveolens, P. radula*	Air, Water, Venus.	**Lovers**	2 of Cups
27	Ginger *Zingiber officinale*	Fire, Water, Mars, Aries, Scorpio.	**Emperor**	2 of Wands
28	Honeysuckle *Lonicera caprifolium*	Water, Moon, Neptune, Cancer, Pisces.	**Moon**	—
29	Hyssop *Hyssopus officinalis*	Fire, Jupiter, Sagittarius.	**Temperance**	Prince of Wands
30	Jasmine *Jasminum grandiflorum*	Water, Moon, Taurus, Cancer.	**High Priestess**	—
31	Juniper Berry *Juniperus communis*	Fire, Sun, Leo.	**Strength**	3 of Pentacles
32	Labdanum (Rock rose) *Cistus ladaniferus*	Water, Moon, Cancer, Scorpio.	**Chariot**	King of Cups
33	Lavender (or Lavandin, Spike) *Lavendula officinalis*	Air, Mercury, Venus, Gemini, Libra.	**Lovers**	9 of Swords
34	Lemon *Citrus limonum*	Water, Moon, Cancer.	**High Priestess**	3 of Cups
35	Lemongrass *Cymbopogon citratus*	Air, Mercury, Gemini.	**Magician**	Ace of Swords
36	Lime *Citrus aurantifolia*	Air, Sun, Aquarius.	**Star**	—
37	Mandarin (or Tangerine) *Citrus reticulata or C. nobilis*	Fire, Sun, Leo.	**Sun**	6 of Cups
38	Marjoram *Origanum majorana, Marjorana hortensis*	Water, Air, Venus, Pisces, Libra.	**Moon**	5 of Cups

MASTER CHART OF THE ESSENTIAL OILS (continued)

	Essential Oils	Astrological Associations	Major Arcana	Minor Arcana
39	Melissa (Lemon Balm) *Melissa officinalis*	Water, Jupiter, Neptune, Pisces.	**Moon**	—
40	Mugwort *Artemisia vulgaris*	Water, Moon, Neptune, Pisces.	**Hanged One**	7 of Cups
41	Myrrh *Commiphora myrrha*	Water, Moon, Saturn, Neptune, Pisces.	**Hanged One**	3 of Swords
42	Myrtle *Myrtus communis*	Earth, Air, Venus, Taurus, Libra.	**Justice**	4 of Wands
43	Narcissus *Narcissus spp., N. poeticus*	Earth, Mercury, Virgo	**Hermit**	—
44	Neroli (or Orange) *Citrus aurantinum bigarada (or Citrus aurantium)*	Fire, Sun, Leo.	**Strength**	—
45	Niaouli (or Cajeput & M.Q.V.) *Melaleuca viridiflora*	Air, Uranus, Libra, Aquarius.	**Fool**	Queen of Swords
46	Nutmeg *Myristica fragrans*	Fire, Jupiter, Sagittarius.	**Wheel of Fortune**	2 of Pentacles
47	Oakmoss *Evernia prunastri*	Earth, Venus, Saturn, Taurus, Capricorn.	**World**	Prince of Pentacles
48	Opoponax *Commiphora erythraea*	Water, Pluto, Scorpio.	**Death**	—
49	Palmarosa *Cymbopogon martinii*	Air, Venus, Libra.	**Justice**	2 of Swords
50	Patchouli *Pogostemon cablin, P. patchouli*	Earth, Venus, Saturn, Taurus, Capricorn.	**Devil**	4 of Pentacles
51	Pennyroyal *Mentha pulegium or Hedeoma pulegioides*	Fire, Water, Mars, Pluto, Scorpio.	**Judgement**	7 of Wands
52	Peppermint *Mentha piperita*	Air, Mercury, Gemini.	**Lovers**	5 of Swords
53	Petitgrain *Citrus bigaradia*	Fire, Mars, Aries.	**Emperor**	8 of Pentacles
54	Pine *Pinus species*	Air, Mars, Aries, Scorpio.	**Tower**	5 of Wands

MASTER CHART OF THE ESSENTIAL OILS (continued)

	Essential Oils	Astrological Associations	Major Arcana	Minor Arcana
55	Rose *Rosa damascena, centifolia or gallica*	Air, Earth, Venus, Taurus, Libra.	**Empress**	—
56	Rosemary *Rosemarinus officinalis*	Fire, Sun, Leo.	**Strength**	Queen of Wands
57	Rue *Ruta graveolens*	Fire, Mars, Aries, Scorpio.	**Death**	10 of Swords
58	Saffron *Crocus sativum*	Fire, Jupiter, Leo, Sagittarius.	**Wheel of Fortune**	—
59	Sage *Salvia officinalis*	Air, Earth, Mercury, Jupiter, Sagittarius.	**Hermit**	10 of Wands
60	Sandalwood (Mysore) *Santalum album*	Water, Venus, Jupiter, Neptune, Pisces.	**Moon**	9 of Cups
61	Sassafras *Sassafras albidum*	Fire, Mars, Aries.	**Tower**	Princess of Wands
62	Spearmint *Mentha spicata*	Air, Mercury, Gemini, Libra.	**Justice**	9 of Pentacles
63	Spikenard (Nard or Valerian) *Nardostachys jatamansi*	Water, Earth, Saturn, Neptune, Virgo, Capricorn.	**Hanged One**	8 of Cups
64	Storax (or Benzoin) *Liquidambar orientalis or syraciflua (or Styrax benzoin, S. tonkinense)*	Air, Mercury, Gemini.	**Magician**	Princess of Swords
65	Thyme (or Linalol) *Thymus vulgaris*	Earth, Venus, Mercury Taurus, Libra.	**Hierophant**	5 of Pentacles
66	Valerian *Valerian officinalis*	Water, Pluto, Scorpio.	**Death**	—
67	Vetiveria zizannoides *Vanilla planifolia (or Myroxylon balsamum)*	Water, Earth, Venus, Taurus, Pisces.	**Empress**	Princess of Cups
68	Vetivert *Vetiveria zizannoides*	Earth, Venus, Saturn, Capricorn.	**World**	Ace of Pentacles
69	Wintergreen (Birch) *Gaultheria procumbens*	Earth, Mercury, Virgo.	**Hermit**	8 of Wands
70	Ylang ylang *Canaga odorata*	Water, Venus, Pisces.	**Empress**	Queen of Cups

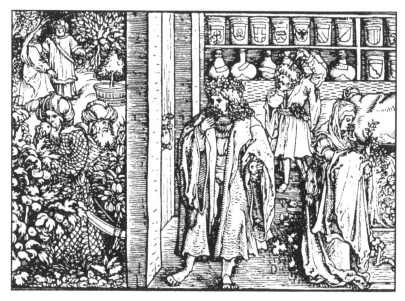

Indoor and outdoor uses of herbs. From Das Kreuterbuch oder Herbarius.

Notes

Chapter 1—Essential Oils

1. Edwin T. Morris, *Fragrance: The Story of Perfume from Cleopatra to Chanel*, p. xiv.

2. Diane Ackerman, *A Natural History of the Senses*, p. 9.

3. Franz Hartmann, *The Metaphysical Properties and Curative Powers of Plants*, p. 12.

4. Often two grades of essential oils are offered, "pure, natural" and "therapeutic." The latter is required only for pharmacological and medical purposes. Either may be used for the purposes of this book.

5. Marcia Barinaga, "How the Nose Knows: Olfactory Receptor Cloned," pp. 209–210.

6. Diane Ackerman, *A Natural History of the Senses*, p. 11.

7. Ibid., p. 20.

Chapter 2—A Magical History of Oils

1. See D. M. Stoddart, "Human Odour Culture: A Zoological Perspective," in Van Toller and Dodd.

2. Magical Magpie, "A Brief History of the Magical and Religious Uses of Perfume and Incense."

3. M. W. Blackden, *Ritual of the Mystery of the Judgment of the Soul*, p. 4.

4. Florence Farr, *Egyptian Magic*.

5. Actually *Kyphi* contained at least sixteen ingredients. See Scott Cunningham's recipes in *The Magic of Incense, Oils, and Brews*, p. 48.

6. Frederic Lees, "Isis Worship in Paris."

7. Theodore H. Gaster, *Myth, Legend, and Custom in the Old Testament*, p. 566.

8. Henna flowers.

9. Song of Solomon (1: 11–14). Note that En Gedi was the site of Cleopatra's perfume manufactory several hundred years later.

10. Victoria Edwards, "Spikenard . . . The Anointing Oil."

11. Mark Haeffner, *The Dictionary of Alchemy*, p. 169.

12. Barbara G. Walker, *The Woman's Dictionary of Symbols and Sacred Objects*, p. 427.

13. Homer, *The Iliad*, XIV 170–174.

14. Julia Lawless, *The Encyclopaedia of Essential Oils*, p. 14.

15. Nik Douglas and Penny Singer, *Sexual Secrets*, p. 102.

16. Edwin T. Morris, *Fragrance*, p. 116.

17. Ibid., p. 118.

18. See Kiyoko Morita, *The Book of Incense*.

19. Thanks to the Shoyeido Corp., purveyors of traditional Japanese Incense since 1705. In the US: Shoyeido USA Inc., 1700 38th Street, Boulder, CO 80301, *shoyeido.com*.

20. Maria Leach, ed., *Funk & Wagnalls Standard Dictionary of Folklore, Mythology, and Legend*, p. 857.

21. Diane Ackerman, *A Natural History of the Senses*, p. 6.

22. Sapere Aude (William Wynn Westcott), *The Science of Alchymy*, p. 19.

23. Frater Albertus, *The Alchemist's Handbook*, p. 16.

24. Ibid., p. 18.

25. Ibid.

26. Manly P. Hall, *The Secret Teachings of All Ages*, p. CXII.

27. Florence Farr (ed.), *Euphrates, Or the Waters of the East* by Eugenius Philalethes.

Chapter 3—About the Tarot

1. Quoted by D. M. Stoddart in "Human Odour Culture: A Zoological Perspective," in Van Toller and Dodd, p. 5.

2. *The Herbal Tarot* and a descriptive book by herbalists Candice Cantin and Michael Tierra are published by U.S. Games Systems Inc.

3. Sheryl Karas, *The Solstice Evergreen*, pp. 10–11.

4. Florence Farr, *Euphrates or the Waters of the East by Eugenius Philalethes.*

Chapter 4—Imagination and Aroma Imaging

1. Cynthia Giles, *The Tarot: History, Mystery, and Lore*, pp. 161–163.

2. Walter J. Freeman, "The Physiology of Perception," p. 78. Freeman's excellent article is a vital resource for anyone interested in applying chaos theory to magic or in theories of olfaction.

3. Ibid., p. 81.

4. Ibid., p. 83.

5. Ibid., p. 85.

6. Edwin T. Morris, *Fragrance*, p. 266.

7. See Cynthia Giles, *The Tarot: History, Mystery, and Lore*, pp. ix–x

8. Valerie Ann Worwood, *Aromantics*, pp. 28–29.

9. E. E. Rehmus, *The Magician's Dictionary*, p. 233. (See also Arthur Versluis, *The Philosophy of Magic*, pp. 35–46.)

10. Ibid.

Chapter 5—The Tarot Oils

1. Some essential oils are recommended by doctors and therapists for internal use (especially in England and France), but you must be sure of your source and method of extraction (for instance, that no toxic chemicals were used in the process), and they should only be so used when directed by a knowledgeable professional.

2. If you have ever had an epileptic seizure, are pregnant, or are very allergic or sensitive, then please research the oils carefully before using. See especially Robert Tisserand's *Essential Oil Safety Data Manual* or Julia Lawless's *The Encyclopaedia of Essential Oils*.

3. If you were to purchase only two expensive oils, I would recommend a good jasmine and rose. Only one or two milliliters are necessary, because they are so highly concentrated. A tiny bit of these two oils goes a long way; too much is overpowering.

4. See previous footnote.

5. Quoted from Willis Barnstone, ed., *The Other Bible* (San Francisco: Harper & Row, 1984), p. 68, in Barbara G. Walker, *The Woman's Dictionary of Symbols and Sacred Objects*, p. 433.

6. See Kathi Keville's *Aromatherapy Notes*.

7. Walker, p. 445.

8. Hakim Moinuddin Chishti, *The Book of Sufi Healing*, p. 61.

Chapter 6—Magic and Ritual

1. Attributed to Dion Fortune.

2. See Kay Turner, "Contemporary Feminist Rituals."

3. Starhawk's book *The Spiral Dance* is a good place to learn about creating Pagan- or Wiccan-style rituals. For ceremonial magic, see any of the books by William Gray; *Techniques of High Magic: A Guide to Self-Empowerment*, by Francis King and Stephen Skinner; or *The Ritual Magic Workbook*, by Dolores Ashcroft-Nowicki.

4. There is a difference between invoking and evoking. Invoking is calling down (usually a "higher power") from another place into your presence. Evoking is calling forth, as in calling the essence to come forth from within.

5. David Howes, "New Guinea: An Olfactory Ethnography."

6. Kathleen Raine, *Yeats, the Tarot, and the Golden Dawn*, p. 46.

7. See Frater Albertus, *The Alchemist's Handbook*.

8. See Valerie Worwood's *Aromantics* for many more wise insights into scent, sex, and attraction.

Chapter 7—Tarot Oil Techniques

1. Monika Jünneman, *Enchanting Scents,* p. 14.

2. If you practice ceremonial magic, Chris Zalewski, in *Herbs in Magic and Alchemy,* describes a Golden Dawn technique for plant communication.

3. Hakim Moinuddin Chishti, *The Book of Sufi Healing,* p. 119.

4. See *The Candle Magick Workbook,* by Kala and Ketz Pajeon, for everything you ever wanted to know about this topic, presented with practicality and sensitivity.

5. Thanks to Alaina Zachary of Malden Bridge, NY, who first taught me this technique.

6. More information on writing affirmations can be found in Shakti Gawain's classic book *Creative Visualization.*

7. The Greek word *kosmein,* from which we get cosmetic, means not only "to decorate" but also "to harmonize."

Bibliography

Ackerman, Diane. *A Natural History of the Senses*. New York: Random House, 1991.

Albertus, Frater. *The Alchemist's Handbook*. York Beach, ME: Samuel Weiser, 1974.

Arctander, Steffen. *Perfume and Flavor Materials of Natural Origin*. Elizabeth, NJ: self-published, 1960.

Ashcroft-Nowicki, Dolores. *The Ritual Magic Workbook*. Wellingborough, Northamptonshire, UK: Aquarian Press, 1986.

Atchley, E. G. Cuthbert F. *A History of the Use of Incense in Divine Worship*, London: Longmans, Green and Co., 1909.

Barinaga, Marcia. "How the Nose Knows: Olfactory Receptor Cloned." *Science* 252, 1991: 209–210.

Blackden, M. W. *Ritual of the Mystery of the Judgment of the Soul*. Edmonds, WA: The Alexandrian Press, n.d.; rpt. 1988.

Blake, William. *Milton, a Poem in Two Books*. London, England: n.p., 1804.

Cantin, Candice, and Michael Tierra. *The Herbal Tarot*. Stamford, CT: U.S. Games, 1988.

Chishti, Hakim Moinuddin. *The Book of Sufi Healing*. Rochester, VT: Inner Traditions, 1991.

Clifford, F. S. *A Romance of Perfume Lands, or, the Search for Capt. Jacob Cole with Interesting Facts about Perfumes and Articles Used in the Toilet*. Boston: Clifford & Co., 1881.

Coats, Alice M. *Flowers and Their Histories*. New York: McGraw-Hill, 1956, 1968.

Crowley, Aleister. *Liber 777: Revised Edition*. Many editions, including free online.

Culpeper, Nicholas. *Culpeper's Complete Herbal and English Physician Enlarged*. Glenwood, IL: Meyerbooks, rpt. 1987.

Cunningham, Scott. *Magical Herbalism: The Secret Craft of the Wise*. St. Paul, MN: Llewellyn, 1982.

———. *The Magic of Incense, Oils, and Brews: A Guide to Their Preparation and Use*. St. Paul, MN: Llewellyn, 1986.

———. *Magical Aromatherapy*. St. Paul, MN: Llewellyn, 1990.

Davis, Patricia. *Aromatherapy: An A–Z*. Saffron Walden, UK: C. W. Daniel, 1988.

———. *Subtle Aromatherapy*. Saffron Walden, UK: C. W. Daniel, 1991.

de Claremont, Lewis. *Legends of Incense, Herb and Oil Magic*. Arlington, TX: Dorene, 1938; rpt 1966.

Donato, Giuseppe, and Monique Seefried. *The Fragrant Past: Perfumes of Cleopatra and Julius Caesar*. Rome: Institute Poligrafico e Zecca dello Stato, 1989.

Douglas, Nik, and Penny Singer. *Sexual Secrets*. New York: Destiny Books, 1979.

Edwards, Victoria. "Spikenard . . . The Anointing Oil." *Common Scents* 1:2, 1989.

———. "Are Synthetic and Natural Oils Identical? An Anthroposophical Approach." *The International Journal of Aromatherapy* 2:2, Summer 1989.

Engen, Trygg. *Odor Sensation and Memory*. New York: Praeger, 1991.

Farr, Florence, ed. *Euphrates or the Waters of the East by Eugenius Philalethes*. 1655. With a commentary by S.S.D.D. Collectanea Hermetica. London: Theosophical Publishing Society, 1896.

Farr, Florence. *Egyptian Magic*. Wellingborough, Northamptonshire, UK: Aquarian, rpt. 1982.

Fischer-Rizzi, Susanne. *Complete Aromatherapy Handbook: Essential Oils for Radiant Health*. New York: Sterling, 1990.

Freeman, Walter J. "The Physiology of Perception." *Scientific American*, Feb. 1991: 78–85.

Gaster, Theodor H. *Myth, Legend, and Custom in the Old Testament: A Comparative Study with Chapters from Sir James G. Frazer's Folklore in the Old Testament*. New York: Harper and Row, 1969.

Gawain, Shakti. *Creative Visualization*. Mill Valley, CA: Whatever Publishing Co., 1978. (See also Bantam, and New World Library.)

Genders, Roy. *Perfume through the Ages.* New York: G. P. Putnam's Sons, 1972.

Gibbons, Boyd. "The Intimate Sense of Smell." *National Geographic,* Sept. 1986: 324–360.

Giles, Cynthia. *The Tarot: History, Mystery, and Lore.* New York: Paragon House, 1992.

Greer, Mary K. *Tarot Mirrors: Reflections of Personal Meaning.* North Hollywood, CA: Newcastle, 1988.

———. *An Audio Exploration of Tarot.* Los Angeles: Audio Renaissance Tapes, 1988.

———. *Tarot for Your Self: A Workbook for the Inward Journey.* Newburyport, MA: Weiser Books, 2019.

———. *Archetypal Tarot: What Your Birth Card Reveals about Your Personality, Your Path, and Your Potential.* Newburyport, MA: Weiser Books, 2021.

Groom, Nigel. *Frankincense and Myrrh: A Study of the Arabian Incense Trade.* London & New York: Longman, 1981.

Gurudas. *Flower Essences and Vibrational Healing.* San Rafael, CA: Cassandra, 1983.

Haeffner, Mark. *The Dictionary of Alchemy: From Maria Prophetissa to Isaac Newton.* London: Aquarian, 1991.

Hall, Manly P. *The Secret Teachings of All Ages: An Encyclopedic Outline of Masonic, Hermetic, Qabbalistic and Rosicrucian Symbolical Philosophy.* Los Angeles: The Philosophical Research Society, 1928, 1988.

Hartmann, Franz. *The Metaphysical Properties and Curative Powers of Plants.* Edmonds, WA: Sure Fire Press, n.d.; rpt. 1990.

Howes, David. "New Guinea: An Olfactory Ethnography." *Dragoco Report* 2, 1992: 71–81.

Jünemann, Monika. *Enchanting Scents.* Wilmot, WI: Lotus Light, 1988.

Karas, Sheryl. *The Solstice Evergreen: History, Folklore and Origins of the Christmas Tree.* Boulder Creek, CA: Aslan, 1991.

Keller, Erich. *The Complete Home Guide to Aromatherapy: Self-Help with Essential Oils.* Tiburon, CA: H. J. Kramer, 1991.

Keville, Kathi. "Essential Oils: Common Sense about Scents." *Vegetarian Times*, 45: 1981.

———. *Aromatherapy Notes.* Nevada City, CA: Oak Valley Herb Farm, 1990, 1992.

King, Francis, and Stephen Skinner. *Techniques of High Magic: A Guide to Self-Empowerment.* Rochester, VT: Destiny, 1976, 1991.

Kull, A. Stoddard. *Secrets of Flowers.* Brattleboro, VT: Stephen Greene, 1969.

Lawless, Julia. *The Encyclopaedia of Essential Oils: The Complete Guide to the Use of Aromatics in Aromatherapy, Herbalism, Health, and Well-Being.* Shaftesbury, UK: Element, 1992.

Leach, Maria, ed. *Funk & Wagnalls Standard Dictionary of Folklore, Mythology, and Legend.* San Francisco: Harper and Row, 1972.

Lees, Frederic. "Isis Worship in Paris: Conversations with the Hierophant Rameses and the High Priestess Anari." *The Humanitarian* XVI:2, 1900.

Lehane, Brendan. *The Power of Plants.* New York: McGraw-Hill, 1977.

Magpie, Magical. "A Brief History of the Magical and Religious Uses of Perfume and Incense." *Green Egg* XXV:28, 1992: 19.

Maple, Eric. *The Secret Lore of Plants and Flowers.* London: Robert Hale, 1980.

Maury, Marguerite. *Marguerite Maury's Guide to Aromatherapy: The Secret of Life and Youth.* Saffron Waldon, UK: C. W. Daniel, 1989.

Morita, Kiyoko. *The Book of Incense: Enjoying the Traditional Art of Japanese Scents.* Tokyo: Kodansha International, 1992.

Morris, Edwin T. *Fragrance: The Story of Perfume from Cleopatra to Chanel.* New York: Charles Scribner's Sons, 1984.

"No One's Sniffing at Aroma Research Now." *Business Week*, Dec. 23, 1991: 82–83.

Pajeon, Kala, and Ketz Pajeon. *The Candle Magic Workbook.* New York: Citadel Press, 1991.

Poucher, William A. *Perfumes, Cosmetics, and Soaps: Being a Treatise on the Production, Manufacture and Application of Perfumes of All Types.* London: Chapman & Hall, 1936.

Raine, Kathleen. *Yeats, the Tarot, and the Golden Dawn.* Dublin: Dolmen Press, 1976.

Rehmus, E. E. *The Magician's Dictionary.* Los Angeles: Feral House, 1990.

Riva, Anna. *The Modern Herbal Spellbook: The Magical Uses of Herbs.* Toluca Lake, CA: International Imports, 1974.

Robbins, Tom. *Jitterbug Perfume.* New York: Bantam, 1984.

Rose, Jeanne. *The Aromatherapy Book: Applications and Inhalations.* Berkeley: North Atlantic Books, 1992.

Sapere Aude (William Wynn Westcott). *The Science of Alchymy: Spiritual and Material.* Edmonds, WA: The Alchemical Press, n.d.; rpt. 1983.

Starck, Marcia. *Earth Mother Astrology: Ancient Healing Wisdom.* St. Paul, MN: Llewellyn, 1989.

Starhawk. *The Spiral Dance: A Rebirth of the Ancient Religion of the Great Goddess.* San Francisco: Harper & Row, 1979.

Steele, John J. "The Nectar of Gaia." *Perfume and Flavorist* 15, July/Aug. 1900: 19–22.

Synnot, Anthony. "A Sociology of Smell." *Canadian Review of Sociology and Anthropology,* 28:4, 1991, 437–459.

Thompson, C. J. S. *The Mystery and Lure of Perfume.* London: John Lane The Bodley Head, 1927.

Tisserand, Robert B. *The Art of Aromatherapy: The Healing and Beautifying Properties of the Essential Oils of Flowers and Herbs.* Rochester, VT: Healing Arts Press, 1977.

Turner, Kay. "Contemporary Feminist Rituals." *The Politics of Women Spirituality: Essays on the Rise of Spiritual Power within the Feminist Movement.* Ed. Charlene Spretnak. Garden City, NY: Anchor, 1982, pp. 219–233.

Valnet, Jean. *The Practice of Aromatherapy: A Classic Compendium of Plant Medicines and Their Healing Properties.* Rochester VT: Healing Arts Press, 1980, 1990.

Van Toller, Steve, and George H. Dodd, eds. *Perfumery: The Psychology and Biology of Fragrance.* London and New York: Chapman and Hall, 1988.

Versluis, Arthur. *The Philosophy of Magic.* Boston & London: Arkana, 1986.

Walker, Barbara G. *The Woman's Dictionary of Symbols and Sacred Objects.* San Francisco: Harper & Row, 1988.

Weisenthal, Debra Balke. "What the Nose Knows." *Vegetarian Times* 182: Oct., 1992: 95–101.

Winter, Ruth. *The Smell Book: Scents, Sex, and Society.* Philadelphia & New York: J. B. Lippincott, 1976.

Worwood, Valerie Ann. *Aromantics.* London: Pan, 1987.

Zalewski, C. L. *Herbs in Magic and Alchemy: Techniques from Ancient Herbal Lore.* Lindfield, NSW: Unity Press, 1990.